THE M.A.X. MUSCLE PLAN 2.0

SECOND EDITION

BRAD SCHOENFELD, PhD

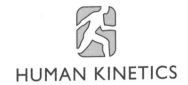

HUMAN KINETICS

MW00354903

Library of Congress Cataloging-in-Publication Data

Names: Schoenfeld, Brad, 1962- author.
Title: The M.A.X. muscle plan 2.0 / Brad Schoenfeld.
Description: Second edition. | Champaign, IL : Human Kinetics, 2022. |
  Includes bibliographical references.
Identifiers: LCCN 2021010385 (print) | LCCN 2021010386 (ebook) | ISBN
  9781718207141 (paperback) | ISBN 9781718207158 (epub) | ISBN
  9781718207165 (pdf)
Subjects: LCSH: Bodybuilding. | Muscle strength.
Classification: LCC GV546.5 .S36 2022 (print) | LCC GV546.5 (ebook) |
  DDC 613.7/13--dc23
LC record available at https://lccn.loc.gov/2021010385
LC ebook record available at https://lccn.loc.gov/2021010386

ISBN: 978-1-7182-0714-1 (print)

Copyright © 2022, 2013 by Brad Schoenfeld

Human Kinetics supports copyright. Copyright fuels scientific and artistic endeavor, encourages authors to create new works, and promotes free speech. Thank you for buying an authorized edition of this work and for complying with copyright laws by not reproducing, scanning, or distributing any part of it in any form without written permission from the publisher. You are supporting authors and allowing Human Kinetics to continue to publish works that increase the knowledge, enhance the performance, and improve the lives of people all over the world.

To report suspected copyright infringement of content published by Human Kinetics, contact us at **permissions@hkusa.com**. To request permission to legally reuse content published by Human Kinetics, please refer to the information at **https://US.HumanKinetics.com/pages/permissions-information**.

This publication is written and published to provide accurate and authoritative information relevant to the subject matter presented. It is published and sold with the understanding that the author and publisher are not engaged in rendering legal, medical, or other professional services by reason of their authorship or publication of this work. If medical or other expert assistance is required, the services of a competent professional person should be sought.

The web addresses cited in this text were current as of April 2021, unless otherwise noted.

Senior Acquisitions Editor: Roger W. Earle; **Managing Editor:** Hannah Werner; **Copyeditor:** Michelle Horn; **Permissions Manager:** Martha Gullo; **Graphic Designer:** Denise Lowry; **Cover Designer:** Keri Evans; **Cover Design Specialist:** Susan Rothermel Allen; **Photograph (cover):** OlegUsmanov/iStock/Getty Images Plus; **Photographs (interior):** Neil Bernstein and Doug Fink; Photos on page 126 by Bret Contreras; **Photo Production Manager:** Jason Allen; **Senior Art Manager:** Kelly Hendren; **Illustrations:** © Human Kinetics; **Printer:** Sheridan Books

We thank Adrenaline Gym in Peekskill, New York, for assistance in providing the location for the photo shoot for this book.

Human Kinetics books are available at special discounts for bulk purchase. Special editions or book excerpts can also be created to specification. For details, contact the Special Sales Manager at Human Kinetics.

Printed in the United States of America   10 9 8 7 6 5 4 3 2 1

The paper in this book is certified under a sustainable forestry program.

Human Kinetics
1607 N. Market Street
Champaign, IL 61820
USA

United States and International
Website: **US.HumanKinetics.com**
Email: info@hkusa.com
Phone: 1-800-747-4457

Canada
Website: **Canada.HumanKinetics.com**
Email: info@hkcanada.com

E8345

Tell us what you think!
Human Kinetics would love to hear what we can do to improve the customer experience. Use this QR code to take our brief survey.

*This book is dedicated to the memory of John Meadows.
A legendary bodybuilder, true gentleman, and great friend;
your impact on the field will be everlasting. RIP.*

CONTENTS

EXERCISE FINDER

EXERCISE	PRIMARY MUSCLES WORKED	OTHER MUSCLES WORKED	SINGLE JOINT OR MULTI-JOINT	PAGE
CHAPTER 3: EXERCISES FOR THE BACK, CHEST, AND ABDOMEN				
BACK				
Dumbbell pullover	lats, sternal pectorals		Single	34
Dumbbell one-arm row	back muscles		Multi	35
T-bar row	back muscles		Multi	36
Barbell reverse-grip bent row	back muscles		Multi	37
Barbell overhand bent row	back muscles		Multi	38
Machine close-grip seated row	back muscles		Multi	39
Machine wide-grip seated row	posterior delts, back muscles		Multi	40
Cable seated row	back muscles		Multi	41
Cable wide-grip seated row	posterior delts, back muscles		Multi	42
Cable one-arm standing low row	back muscles		Multi	43
Chin-up	back muscles	biceps	Multi	44
Pull-up	back muscles		Multi	45
Lat pull-down	back muscles		Multi	46
Neutral-grip lat pull-down	back muscles		Multi	47
Reverse-grip lat pull-down	back muscles		Multi	48
Cable straight-arm lat pull-down	back muscles		Single	49
Cross cable lat pull-down	back muscles		Multi	50
CHEST				
Dumbbell incline press	upper pectorals, triceps, front delts		Multi	51

EXERCISE	PRIMARY MUSCLES WORKED	OTHER MUSCLES WORKED	SINGLE JOINT OR MULTI-JOINT	PAGE
Dumbbell decline press	lower aspect of the sternal pectorals, front delts, triceps		Multi	52
Dumbbell chest press	sternal pectorals	front delts, triceps	Multi	53
Barbell incline press	upper pectorals, triceps, front delts		Multi	54
Barbell chest press	sternal pectorals, triceps, front delts		Multi	55
Barbell decline press	lower aspect of the sternal pectorals, triceps, front delts		Multi	56
Machine incline press	upper pectorals	front delts, triceps	Multi	57
Machine chest press	sternal pectorals	front delts, triceps	Multi	58
Dumbbell flat fly	sternal pectorals	front delts	Single	59
Dumbbell incline fly	upper pectorals	front delts	Single	60
Pec deck fly	sternal pectorals	front delts	Single	61
Cable fly	sternal pectorals	front delts	Single	62
Chest dip	lower aspect of the sternal pectorals	front delts, triceps	Multi	63
ABDOMEN				
Crunch	upper abdominal region		Multi	64
Reverse crunch	lower abdominal region		Multi	65
Bicycle crunch	abs		Multi	66
Roman chair side crunch	obliques		Multi	67
Stability ball abdominal crunch	abs		Multi	68
Cable rope kneeling crunch	upper portion of the abs		Multi	69
Cable rope kneeling twisting crunch	abs, obliques		Multi	70

EXERCISE	PRIMARY MUSCLES WORKED	OTHER MUSCLES WORKED	SINGLE JOINT OR MULTI-JOINT	PAGE
Dumbbell incline biceps curl	biceps (long head)		Single	93
Dumbbell preacher curl	biceps (short head)		Single	94
Barbell preacher curl	biceps (short head)		Single	95
Machine preacher curl	biceps (short head)		Single	96
Concentration curl	biceps (short head)		Single	97
Dumbbell standing hammer curl	brachialis, brachioradialis, upper arms		Single	98
Barbell curl	biceps		Single	99
Barbell drag curl	biceps (long head)		Single	100
Cable rope hammer curl	brachialis, brachioradialis, upper arms		Single	101
Cable curl	biceps		Single	102
Cable one-arm curl	biceps		Single	103
ARMS (TRICEPS)				
Dumbbell overhead triceps extension	triceps (long head)		Single	104
Cable rope overhead triceps extension	triceps (long head)		Single	105
Skull crusher	triceps		Single	106
Machine skull crusher	triceps		Single	107
Dumbbell triceps kickback	triceps (middle and lateral heads)		Single	108
Cable triceps kickback	triceps (middle and lateral heads)		Single	109
Cable triceps press-down	triceps (middle and lateral heads)		Single	110
Triceps dip	triceps		Single	111
Machine triceps dip	triceps		Single	112

EXERCISE	PRIMARY MUSCLES WORKED	OTHER MUSCLES WORKED	SINGLE JOINT OR MULTI-JOINT	PAGE
CHAPTER 5: EXERCISES FOR THE LOWER BODY				
MULTI-JOINT EXERCISES				
Walking lunge	quads, glutes	hamstrings	Multi	**114**
Barbell lunge	quads, glutes	hamstrings	Multi	**115**
Dumbbell lunge	quads, glutes	hamstrings	Multi	**116**
Dumbbell reverse lunge	quads, glutes	hamstrings	Multi	**117**
Dumbbell side lunge	adductors, all lower body		Multi	**118**
Dumbbell step-up	quads, glutes	hamstrings	Multi	**119**
Barbell front squat	frontal thighs, quads, glutes	hamstrings	Multi	**120**
Barbell back squat	quads, glutes	hamstrings	Multi	**121**
Barbell split squat	quads, glutes	hamstrings	Multi	**122**
Bulgarian squat	quads, glutes	hamstrings	Multi	**123**
Leg press	quads, glutes	hamstrings	Multi	**124**
Deadlift	all lower body	upper-body muscles	Multi	**125**
Barbell hip thrust	glutes	hamstrings	Multi	**126**
SINGLE-JOINT EXERCISES				
Good morning	glutes, hamstrings		Single	**127**
Sissy squat	rectus femoris, quads		Single	**128**
Barbell stiff-legged deadlift	glutes, hamstrings		Single	**129**
Dumbbell stiff-legged deadlift	glutes, hamstrings		Single	**130**
Cable glute kickback	glutes, hamstrings		Single	**131**
Hyperextension	glutes, hamstrings		Single	**132**
Reverse hyperextension	glutes, hamstrings		Single	**133**
Leg extension	quads		Single	**134**
Unilateral leg extension	quads		Single	**135**

EXERCISE	PRIMARY MUSCLES WORKED	OTHER MUSCLES WORKED	SINGLE JOINT OR MULTI-JOINT	PAGE
Lying leg curl	hamstrings		Single	**136**
Machine kneeling leg curl	hamstrings		Single	**137**
Machine seated leg curl	hamstrings		Single	**138**
Toe press	calf muscles (gastrocnemius)		Single	**139**
Machine seated calf raise	calf muscles (soleus)		Single	**140**
Machine standing calf raise	calf muscles (gastrocnemius)		Single	**141**

GUIDE TO MUSCLES

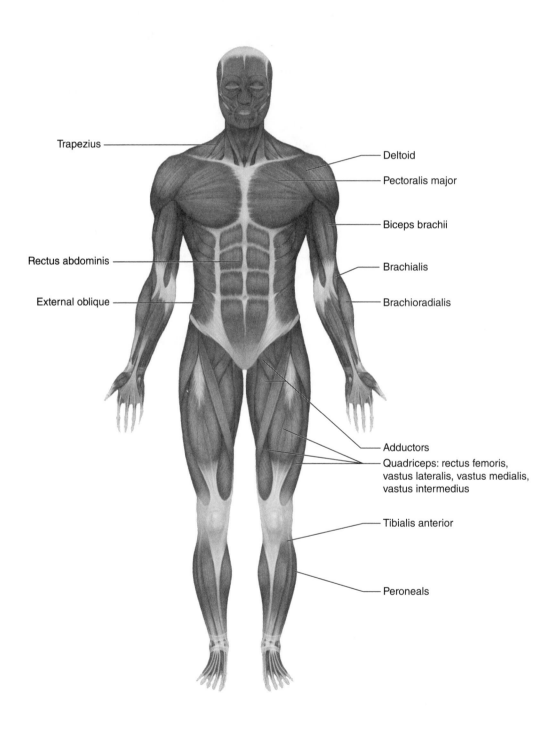

Trapezius

Rectus abdominis

External oblique

Deltoid

Pectoralis major

Biceps brachii

Brachialis

Brachioradialis

Adductors

Quadriceps: rectus femoris,
vastus lateralis, vastus medialis,
vastus intermedius

Tibialis anterior

Peroneals

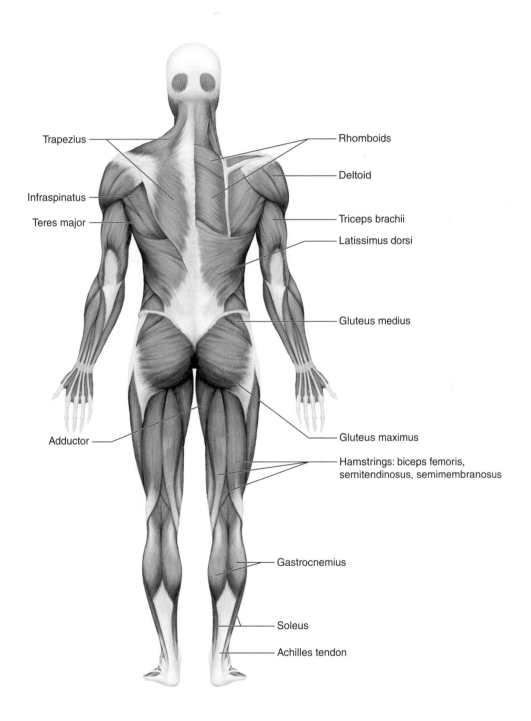

Trapezius

Infraspinatus

Teres major

Adductor

Rhomboids

Deltoid

Triceps brachii

Latissimus dorsi

Gluteus medius

Gluteus maximus

Hamstrings: biceps femoris,
semitendinosus, semimembranosus

Gastrocnemius

Soleus

Achilles tendon

FOREWORD

The year 2012 was one of my best yet scariest years ever. It was then that I ventured out of the comfortable corporate world at JPMorgan Chase and dove full time into the health and fitness industry. I had grown up a bodybuilder and loved to help others, so this transition was exciting but intense because now it was either sink or swim. I was also keenly interested in the science of what makes things happen to our bodies, so now I would have more time to devote to learning. I decided to start my own website and figured that interviewing experts would be a great place to start. With a little fear behind me, I decided I had better knock my interviews out of the park so I wouldn't have to crawl back to the bank and ask for my old job back.

I had been hearing about a guy in New York named Brad Schoenfeld. In fact, I was studying everything he said. I found myself nodding my head as I read his work. It made sense. Much of what I had done had worked in the bodybuilding and nutrition realms, but the truth is, it was more of a gut feeling based on experience than a deep knowledge of the details of why things happen. Brad seemed to be filling in the blanks for me. Oh, this is why this works, this is why this doesn't work, and so on. I reached out to him, hoping he would have time for a quick interview, and he responded with a quick yes. I was ecstatic. We ended up doing two parts because, well, honestly, I just wanted to learn more myself, but the side effect was my website followers got some very advanced knowledge dropped on them.

After the interview, Brad and I kept in touch, and I had begun carrying his paper, "The Mechanisms of Muscle Hypertrophy and Their Application to Resistance Training," around with me like a bible. I read it over, and over, and over. I wasn't the only one. Many bodybuilders I knew started referencing his work. If you know the bodybuilding community, you know we can be a bit of a meathead bunch when it comes to accepting "science" or evidence outside of our own personal experience. Somehow Brad was bridging this gap. I kept noticing more and more of my colleagues popping in and asking Brad questions or sharing his work. It helped that Brad has competed as a bodybuilder himself, but what really helped the most was Brad acknowledging a lot of the good things that bodybuilders had done, and when challenging long-held beliefs, he did it with class and an obvious good intention in his heart. You can search the bodybuilding community high and low and you won't find a single successful person that doesn't respect Brad's work. This is quite remarkable.

Brad eventually asked me to guest lecture to his class, which was absolutely amazing for me because having the respect of someone in his league really meant a great deal. Later, Brad visited, and we trained together and made videos for my YouTube channel that were wildly popular. I am looking forward to doing more of this in the future with him!

You are in for a treat reading this book. Brad is going to teach you how to think about exercise at a high level and at a more detailed level. Simply put, you are going to have the information you need to allow you to build the best program for *you* and learn how to reach your ultimate potential!

Thank you, Brad, for all you do for the community!

John Meadows, CSCS, CISSN
IFBB Pro Bodybuilder

ACKNOWLEDGMENTS

This book was many years in the making, and there are a number of people I would like to thank for helping see it to fruition.

First and foremost, thank you to the editorial staff at Human Kinetics for your diligent efforts in bringing this book to fruition. In particular, I'd like to thank Roger Earle for taking the lead and coordinating all aspects of the publication process. It's always a pleasure to work with such a true professional; there is no better fitness editor in the field. I'd also like to thank Hannah Werner for assuming the project management and proofreading duties and Alexis Koontz for taking charge of marketing; your efforts are greatly appreciated.

To John Meadows: I'm truly honored that you took the time and effort to write the foreword to my book. You serve as a role model in the sport of bodybuilding, epitomizing what can be accomplished when you combine scientific training with practical experience and a supreme drive to be the best!

To my brother, Glenn Schoenfeld: Thank you for facilitating my entrance into the fitness field and helping me when I needed it most. I would not be where I am today without your early support and guidance!

To Bret Contreras and Alan Aragon: Many thanks for your keen eye in reviewing various aspects of the text. You are true friends and great colleagues!

Finally, to my parents: You instilled the importance of the scientific method in me from an early age, and it has shaped who I am in every way. I will love you both through eternity. Rest in peace.

INTRODUCTION

I grew up a skinny kid. To say I was rail-thin would be a gross understatement. For years, it negatively affected my psyche, sapping my self-esteem. I became increasingly self-conscious about my appearance. I was embarrassed to go to the beach in a swimsuit. The psychological impact pervaded all aspects of my life as a teenager.

Everything changed shortly after college when I found bodybuilding.

The iron became my savior. I hit the gym virtually every day like clockwork. Never missed workouts. Traded in junk food for "clean eating." I was determined to bring about a change in my physique and willing to do almost anything necessary to make it happen.

My training and nutritional knowledge was largely derived from the plethora of bodybuilding magazines published at the time. *Muscle & Fitness*, *Flex*, *Iron Man Magazine*, *Muscular Development*, *MuscleMag* . . . I subscribed to them all. When delivery day came, I'd rush out to the mailbox (yes, at that time there were no digital versions!), rip open the plastic packaging, and devour each issue from cover to cover. I created my workout routines based on those of my favorite bodybuilders back in the day. Suffice to say, my approach wasn't very systematic. I'd string together a program of, say, Lee Labrada's chest workout, Tom Platz's quad workout, Lee Haney's back workout, and so on, and perform each set of each exercise exactly as described. Every month or so, I'd switch things up and try out a different bodybuilder's routine for a given muscle group—my unsystematic attempt at employing the Joe Weider concept of "muscle confusion."

On the surface, the approach seemed perfectly logical. After all, I reasoned, pro bodybuilders must know a thing or two about building muscle, right? Who better to emulate when trying to pack on lean mass than guys with 20-inch arms and 30-inch thighs?

Early on, the strategy worked fairly well. I gained appreciable muscle. My self-esteem soared. I actually looked forward to going to the beach. Others took notice; some even asked me to help them with their workouts and nutrition. My journey into a career in fitness had begun.

But after about a year of hard training, I hit the proverbial wall. Results plateaued. No matter which bodybuilder's routine I tried, I couldn't seem to make further progress. Frustration set in. I was at a loss as to what to do.

And then I got the "aha!" moment.

It finally occurred to me that I was going about things all wrong; I couldn't simply follow the routines of the pros and expect to achieve comparable results. Like the vast majority of people, I neither possessed their superior genetics nor indulged in their pharmacology. Over time, I came to understand that my initial results were achieved largely *despite* what I was doing, not because of it.

The fact is, most people can gain muscle by following pretty much any structured resistance training program—at least in the early stages of training. Simply challenge your body beyond its present capacity on a consistent basis and your muscles will adapt by getting bigger. Unfortunately, such an approach takes you only so far. Maximizing your own genetic potential requires adopting a more scientific mindset that individualizes program prescription to your unique needs and abilities.

Ever since that time, I've made it my life's mission to become a fitness educator and promote an evidence-based approach to muscle building. My pursuit compelled me to obtain a master's degree and subsequently a PhD in the field, where my research focused on investigating applied methods for optimizing muscle development. In the process, I competed as a natural bodybuilder and trained numerous high-level physique athletes, including several pros. This combination of research-based knowledge and practical in-the-trenches experience furthered my understanding of the factors that make muscles grow as well as the unique interindividual responses that people have to training. I used my insights to create a systematic method for muscle building that continued to evolve as I gained further knowledge and experience. I employed the method with hundreds of private personal training clients over the years, consistently achieving terrific results. The blueprint of these efforts ultimately became the basis for writing this book.

I penned the first edition of *The M.A.X. Muscle Plan* back in 2011. My goal was to enlighten readers as to the science of muscle development and provide a template for training and nutrition that could be readily adapted to suit individual needs and abilities. The response was overwhelmingly positive. To this day, I continue to receive numerous emails from readers telling me about their success using the program.

However, much has changed since the book's initial publication. A true scientist is constantly reassessing his or her opinions based on emerging evidence, and research conducted over the past decade has impelled me to change my views on various facets of exercise and nutritional programming—in some cases considerably so. Moreover, reader feedback afforded me with insights into aspects of the book that required improvement or clarification. I ultimately realized that the book needed an overhaul to bring it up to current standards and provide the most cutting-edge information on maximizing muscular gains.

After many months of intensive editing, I couldn't be happier with how *The M.A.X. Muscle Plan 2.0* turned out. Here's an overview of what's new.

Several of the chapters have been completely rewritten to best reflect our understanding of the science of muscle building and their relevance to manipulation of program variables and nutritional protocols. Other chapters have somewhat more subtle revisions designed to better reflect my current viewpoints on best training practices and address relevant issues gleaned from feedback on the previous edition. I also added two new chapters: a warm-up chapter (chapter 6) that discusses how to prepare for your workouts and a Q&A chapter (chapter 13) that provides answers to the most frequently asked questions I've received from readers over the years. In all, this edition contains approximately 50 percent new content, substantially improving its practical utility.

In sum, the M.A.X. Muscle Plan isn't just another one-size-fits-all workout program. Rather, it aims to bridge the gap between science and practice, teaching you how to individualize training and nutritional prescription to optimize your own genetic potential. Regardless of whether you're the hardest of hard-gainers or someone who gains muscle relatively easily, this book will help take your physique to the next level; all you need to do is put in the requisite consistent effort.

Enjoy the journey.

THE SCIENCE OF HYPERTROPHY: WHAT MAKES MUSCLES GROW?

The human body is by far the most amazing piece of machinery in the world, capable of incredible feats of strength, creativity, and intellect. Perhaps its most remarkable attribute, though, is its unique ability to adapt to almost any obstacle it faces. No human-made device comes anywhere close to approximating these adaptive qualities.

That said, inherently the body doesn't like change. Under normal circumstances, it strives to maintain a stable state known as homeostasis. Only when subjected to stress is the body forced to deviate from its homeostatic comfort zone and produce an adaptive response. The muscles are no exception. Just like every other body tissue, they seek to maintain homeostasis. Accordingly, muscle growth takes place only when a stress (such as lifting a weight) is imposed that challenges your muscles beyond their present capacity. This concept, called the **principle of overload**, is one of the most important tenets of muscle development; if muscles are not sufficiently challenged on a regular basis, they have no impetus to develop.

Here's how things play out in the gym. When you lift weights in a manner that challenges your muscles, your body perceives the associated stress as a threat to its survival. Your body, in turn, adapts by getting bigger and stronger so that it can effectively deal with the same stimulus if and when it is encountered in the future. This adaptation—muscle development—continues in such a manner as long as you regularly apply physical stressors to overload your muscles.

During the initial stages of training, the primary exercise-related adaptation involves reprogramming your nervous system. Basically, your muscles become more economical at coordinating movement patterns involved in lifting weights. You progress from disorganized, choppy movements to smooth, efficient ones. Over time, your skill level improves until the movements become second nature. This neurological response brings about substantial increases in strength with limited contribution from increases in muscle size.

Once exercise technique becomes more fluent, usually after a couple months of consistent training, you can channel your energies into exerting greater amounts of force during a given lift. At this point your muscles begin to grow larger, facilitating further improvements in strength. Muscle growth is achieved by increases in both the size and number of the contractile proteins (e.g., actin, myosin, etc.) that carry out movement. Contractile proteins are primarily added next to one another in a parallel fashion, like sardines in a tin can. The more contractile proteins you add, the bigger your muscles get.

Muscle growth isn't a one-way street, though; the process can also work in reverse. Muscle is a metabolically active tissue, and its maintenance requires increased caloric expenditure. If you stop working out, your body will perceive unused muscle as energetically wasteful and thus initiate catabolic (breaking down) processes to get rid of the excess; the upshot is a loss of muscle, a.k.a. atrophy. This is known as the **principle of reversibility**, a.k.a. "use it or lose it." Although your body seeks homeostasis, it is actually in a constant state of flux that favors muscle atrophy unless you actively engage in challenging muscular activity on a regular basis.

TRIGGERING MUSCLE GROWTH

When it comes to muscle, proteins are king. Although water makes up the majority of muscle tissue (approximately 70 percent of muscle weight), it's the protein component (approximately 25 percent of muscle weight) that is responsible for carrying out human movement. The extent of muscle development is predicated on the balance between muscle protein synthesis, or building, and muscle protein breakdown. When synthesis is greater than breakdown, you are in an anabolic (building up) state that's conducive to gaining muscle.

Contrary to popular belief, you don't build your muscles while working out. In fact, the opposite actually occurs. Muscle tissue breaks down at an accelerated rate during training, and protein synthesis is largely suppressed. Although this may seem counterintuitive, it is necessary for facilitating bigger, stronger muscles. Compare it to renovating your kitchen. You have to tear out the existing Formica countertops and the pressboard cabinetry before installing the high-end granite and fine hardwood, right? Similarly, outmoded muscle proteins must first be demolished and removed to allow newer, better proteins to take their place.

Muscle tissue rebuilds after exercise. During this time, muscle protein synthesis skyrockets and breakdown gradually diminishes. Protein synthesis can remain elevated for 48 hours or more post-exercise. During this time, your muscles supercompensate by growing larger.

The underlying processes responsible for muscle development are highly complex, and although our understanding of the topic has increased greatly over the past few decades, much still remains undetermined. It is generally accepted that the regulation of muscle tissue is carried out via the signaling of various pathways associated with protein synthesis (anabolic) and breakdown (catabolic). These pathways are diverse and provide a variety of avenues for muscle to adapt to overload. The common element of all muscle-building pathways is that they conduct signals through specialized enzymes, setting off a chain of events that ultimately promotes protein synthesis while inhibiting protein breakdown.

Current theory proposes that three primary mechanisms help to regulate exercise-related muscle growth: mechanical tension, muscle damage, and metabolic stress (15). Although evidence indicates all three mechanisms can promote anabolic effects, the extent to which they are involved remains controversial, and it is not clear whether they are synergistic or become redundant at a given threshold (26). What follows is a brief discussion of these mechanisms and their potential contribution to the hypertrophic response.

1. **Mechanical tension.** Stress, or tension, exerted on muscles during resistance exercise is widely established as the most important factor in muscle development. The forces produced when lifting weights disturbs the integrity of working muscles, thus bringing about a phenomenon called mechanotransduction. Simply stated, mechanotransduction is the process by which mechanical forces are converted into chemical activity, which is facilitated via sensors located at the muscle membrane. As noted above, this sets off an intracellular signaling cascade whereby a series of enzymes ultimately drive the muscle-building process. Numerous anabolic and catabolic pathways have been identified, and their complex interaction ultimately determines the extent of muscle development.

   Intuitively, the importance of mechanical tension would seem to suggest that heavier loads would be superior for muscle building. After all, tension is necessarily higher when lifting heavier, right?

   Well, not necessarily…

   Emerging research indicates that within wide limits, you gain as much muscle from training with relatively light weights as you do from heavier loads (20). Although we can only speculate on the reasons for this phenomenon, a plausible explanation is that mechanical tension inevitably increases as you approach muscle failure. For example, say you are curling a weight that you can lift 20 times (i.e., your 20RM). The first few reps of the lift will be very easy to perform, and thus the tension exerted necessarily will be low. However, as you continue to curl the load, tension will become exceedingly greater as the load gets more and more difficult to lift. By the last few reps, the muscles are under a great deal of tension in their effort to complete the movement.

   Now, there does seem to be a limit to how light you can lift without compromising results. Research has shown that while training at 40% 1RM to failure elicited similar growth as training at 80% 1RM in both the arms and legs, results were substantially compromised when the load was lowered to 20% 1RM (8). This indicates that a minimum threshold of mechanical tension exists to maximize the hypertrophic response, which persists even when training to muscle failure. It should be pointed out that subjects in the study performed an average of more than 60 repetitions at 20% 1RM. That's a lot of reps—more than most lifters would ever perform—thereby calling into question the practical implications of the presence of a minimum threshold.

2. **Muscle damage.** Anyone who lifts weights has undoubtedly felt achy and sore after an intense exercise session. This phenomenon, called delayed-onset muscle soreness (DOMS), generally manifests approximately 24 hours after an intense workout, and the peak effects are seen about two to three days post-exercise. DOMS is initiated by localized damage to muscle tissue in the form of microtears in both the contractile proteins and surface membrane (i.e., sarcolemma) of the working muscles (see the sidebar, What Causes Muscle Soreness After a Workout?, in chapter 6 for additional insights into the mechanisms of DOMS). What many people fail to grasp, however, is that a certain amount of muscle damage may indirectly benefit muscle development (16).

Here's why.

The response to muscle damage can be likened to the acute inflammatory response to infection. Once the body perceives damage, immune cells (neutrophils, macrophages, and so on) migrate to the damaged tissue to remove cellular debris to help maintain the fiber's ultrastructure. In the process, the body produces signaling molecules called cytokines that activate the release of growth factors involved in muscle development. In this roundabout way, localized inflammation—a source of DOMS—conceivably leads to a growth response that, in effect, strengthens the ability of muscle tissue to withstand future muscle damage.

That said, soreness is by no means a prerequisite for muscle development. Your muscles, connective tissue, and immune system become increasingly efficient in dealing with fiber-related damage associated with intense training—a phenomenon called the **repeated bout effect** (again, an adaptive response) (10). Various physiological and structural adaptations that take place gradually reduce the sensation of pain. Generally speaking, the more you train at high levels of intensity, the greater your resistance to muscle soreness—even though you invariably inflict a modest amount of damage to fibers. This is why some of the world's top bodybuilders never get sore after a workout yet display impressive muscularity—and thus why you shouldn't judge the quality of your workout based on the level of DOMS. Furthermore, too much soreness can be detrimental to muscle growth. If you're so sore that it hurts to sit or raise your arms overhead, you've exceeded your body's ability to repair the damaged muscle tissue and train effectively—and that means you're not growing! Thus, it is speculated there may be a "sweet spot" whereby a moderate amount of damage may augment hypertrophy while substantial damage impairs the growth response. The veracity of this hypothesis remains unclear.

3. **Metabolic stress.** Perhaps the most intriguing factor associated with muscle development is exercise-induced metabolic stress. Research on healthy men whose legs were immobilized by a cast demonstrated that daily application of a pressure cuff to their upper thighs, a procedure shown to induce substantial metabolic stress, significantly helped to attenuate muscle wasting, even in the absence of exercise (5). Other studies have found that blood flow restriction (BFR) exercise performed with very light weights—far less than what is normally considered sufficient for promoting muscular adaptations—can promote significant muscle growth, potentially as a result of generating a substantial amount of metabolic stress (9).

The proposed muscle-building effects of metabolic stress conceivably can be attributed to the production of by-products of metabolism called metabolites. These molecular fragments (including lactate, hydrogen ion, and inorganic phosphate, among others) are thought to indirectly mediate cell signaling (26). Metabolic stress is heightened when you train with moderate to higher repetitions; if you've ever "felt the burn" when pumping out a set of 15 reps, this is the result of local metabolite accumulation (i.e., lactic acid).

Some scientists believe that the anabolic effects of metabolic stress are accomplished, at least in part, by increasing water within muscle—a phenomenon known as cell swelling. Studies have shown that cell swelling stimulates protein synthesis and simultaneously decreases protein breakdown (7). It is not clear exactly why cell swelling causes an anabolic effect, but the prevailing theory suggests a self-preservation mechanism. That is, an increase in water within the cell exerts pressure against the cell wall, similar to overinflating a rubber tire. The cell, in turn, perceives this as a threat to its integrity and responds by sending out anabolic signals that initiate strengthening of its ultrastructure.

Understand that mechanical tension, muscle damage, and metabolic stress generally do not exist in isolation. Rather, they interact to varying extents depending on the training scheme and potentially may combine to produce an additive effect on muscle building. That said, you don't have to consciously program the mechanisms into your routine. As we'll discuss, simply manipulating variables across the training cycle will accomplish this goal, ensuring you'll take advantage of any potential benefits obtained from combining mechanisms.

TIME UNDER TENSION

Some fitness pros have put forth the hypothesis that an optimal **time under tension** (TUT) exists for hypertrophy training. Simply stated, TUT is the duration of a set; the longer the set, the higher the TUT. Although TUT recommendations differ somewhat between proponents of the theory, most peg the hypertrophic sweet spot at approximately 30-60 seconds. While the concept of TUT may sound good in theory, the question is, does it have research-based support?

My doctoral dissertation work provides some intriguing insights into the topic. The study investigated muscular adaptations between a bodybuilding-style routine (three sets of 10 reps per exercise) versus a powerlifting-style routine (seven sets of three reps per exercise); the additional sets performed by the powerlifting group equated the total work performed between groups (18). The results: After eight weeks of training, both groups showed similar increases in hypertrophy. Now here's the interesting thing pertaining to TUT. The duration of the sets for the powerlifting group was much shorter compared to the bodybuilding group, which seemingly refutes the concept of an optimal TUT. However, because the powerlifting group performed more than twice as many total sets as the bodybuilding group, the total TUT per exercise was similar over the course of the study. This suggests that the TUT for a given muscle should be viewed in the context of a training session (or perhaps across weekly sessions to account for training frequency) as opposed to the duration of a set. In support of this theory, we carried out a follow-up study that again compared muscle growth in powerlifting- versus bodybuilding-type training; however, as opposed to my dissertation study, both groups performed three sets per exercise. Thus, TUT for each session was substantially higher in the bodybuilding group. At the conclusion of the eight-week training period, results showed that the bodybuilding group achieved greater increases in muscle size compared to the powerlifting group. Although causality cannot be drawn from correlation, the findings of these two studies when taken in combination seem to suggest that per-session TUT is more relevant to hypertrophy than a per-set basis.

Note that training tempo impacts TUT. If you lift slower at a given rep range, then TUT necessarily increases during the set. If an optimal per-set TUT does in fact exist, we'd expect that slower concentric tempos promote greater hypertrophy than faster tempos. However, there is no evidence this is the case when training is carried out with equal levels of effort (19). In fact, performing concentric reps very slowly seems to have somewhat of a detrimental effect on growth (see the Superslow Training sidebar in chapter 2). Moreover, TUT doesn't distinguish between durations of the concentric and eccentric actions. As discussed in chapter 2, evidence shows that the two actions may benefit from different training tempos. Thus, it would seem misguided to calculate TUT as a single value without considering the individual components that compose a repetition.

Bottom line: The concept of an optimal TUT for muscle building is overly simplistic and lacks supporting objective evidence. It's better to focus on total training volume (as discussed in chapter 2); if you do that, achieving a sufficient TUT ultimately will take care of itself.

CALLING ALL SATELLITES

Muscle building is predicated on your body's capacity for protein synthesis; therefore, the relevant machinery must be in place to produce the required muscle proteins. This protein-making machinery is located in the cell nucleus.

Whereas most bodily tissues have only one nucleus, muscle fibers are multinucleated, meaning they contain many nuclei. This should make intuitive sense. Most cells in the body have a fixed size; in most cases, the ability to become larger is counterproductive. Alternatively, muscle needs to be able to grow bigger and stronger in response to imposed demands. As you can imagine, this requires a lot of machinery! Compare it to a factory. If you have only a single processing plant, your capacity to produce a given product is limited to the capacity of that one unit. However, add a second plant and you effectively double your production capacity. Add a couple more plants and you increase production fourfold. The more available plants, the greater your production capacity.

There's one little problem, though . . .

As mentioned, the body doesn't like excess. It wants to maintain homeostasis in the manner that is least taxing. Thus, muscle initially contains only enough nuclei to meet its perceived demands for producing proteins. What happens, then, when you begin a workout regimen and suddenly need additional nuclei to make more proteins? Enter the wonder of satellite cells.

Satellite cells are the muscles' equivalent of stem cells. These nonspecialized cells reside near the muscle fiber and remain dormant unless and until aroused by strenuous exercise, muscle damage, or both. Once stimulated, satellite cells go into action. They multiply in number, become more specialized, and fuse to existing muscle fibers to provide the precursor materials needed for repair and subsequent growth of new muscle tissue. Perhaps more importantly, they donate their nuclei to the working muscle fibers so that protein synthesis can increase and support growth (2, 12). It is believed that once you reach a certain level of muscularity, additional growth cannot occur without the contribution of satellite cells (1).

A study from the University of Alabama highlights just how important satellite cells are in maximizing muscle development. The researchers studied the response of 66 adults to 16 weeks of resistance training that focused on the quadriceps muscles (14). At the end of the study, participants were classified into one of three groups based on the extent of the growth of their quads: extreme responders (average increase of 58 percent in muscle size), moderate responders (average increase of 28 percent in muscle size), and nonresponders (no tangible change in muscle size). While half the participants were considered moderate responders, 25 percent achieved tremendous muscle gains whereas the others failed to improve at all. One of the most striking reasons for these differences was that both extreme and moderate responders displayed far more satellite cell activity (23 and 19 percent, respectively) than nonresponders. This supports the conclusion that satellite cells are a limiting factor in muscle development and that increasing their activity stimulates greater growth.

THE HORMONE CONNECTION

The endocrine glands secrete hormones into the bloodstream and these substances subsequently interact with target tissues to regulate physiological processes. Although numerous hormones exist, several are specific to carrying out anabolic actions that help to drive muscle development. The three most widely studied hormones are testosterone, insulin-like growth factor-1, and growth hormone.

1. **Testosterone.** Widely regarded as the king of all muscle-building hormones, testosterone promotes muscle growth in a variety of ways. First, it directly increases protein synthesis and inhibits protein breakdown (24, 27). Second, it activates satellite cells, facilitating their effects on muscle tissue (4, 22). Finally, it can indirectly contribute to protein accretion by stimulating the release of other hormones involved in anabolism (21). Although these anabolic effects are seen in the absence of exercise, lifting weights magnifies the actions of testosterone. In males, the majority of testosterone is produced in the testes. Women produce only a small fraction of the testosterone of the average male, which is a primary reason why most women find it difficult to bulk up.

2. **Insulin-like growth factor-1.** Although testosterone gets most of the publicity when it comes to building muscle, insulin-like growth factor-1 (IGF-1) has been identified as a potentially important player in exercise-induced hypertrophy as well. As the name implies, IGF-1 has a similar molecular structure to that of insulin. Several types of IGF-1 have been identified. The systemic form, produced primarily in the liver, is stimulated by growth hormone (GH) and, upon its release, promotes anabolic effects in target tissues including muscle (23). In addition, a muscle-specific form called mechano growth factor (MGF), activated in response to muscle contraction, is proposed to be particularly relevant to muscle adaptation. Since MGF is secreted locally within the muscle—not into the bloodstream—it doesn't qualify as a hormone; MGF therefore will be discussed in the next section covering myokines.

3. **Growth hormone.** Despite its name, growth hormone (GH) is not nearly as anabolic as either IGF-1 or testosterone. GH is primarily a repartitioning agent. It is involved in increasing the use of fat for fuel as well as stimulating the uptake and incorporation of amino acids into various body proteins. Contrary to popular belief, GH seems to have a greater effect on reducing body fat than on building muscle. As previously mentioned, most of the anabolic effects of GH are likely related to its

symbiotic relationship with IGF-1 (25). Specifically, GH preferentially upregulates the production of IGF-1, including the MGF form. Given the proposed actions of IGF-1 in exercise-induced hypertrophy, this may be the most prominent muscle-building role of GH.

It doesn't take an exercise scientist to realize that hormones play a substantial role in muscle development. Compare the physique of a juiced-up pro bodybuilder with that of someone who competes naturally, and the amount of influence that anabolic hormones can have on muscle size becomes patently apparent. It is not unusual for a person to gain 20-30 pounds (10-14 kg) in a matter of weeks after going on a steroid cycle. Good luck if you try gaining that naturally.

Interestingly, research shows that intense resistance exercise can cause large hormonal spikes after training. In some cases, increases in certain hormone levels are of the magnitude of several hundred percent. It therefore seems to make sense that the best exercise routines for muscle growth are those that produce the greatest hormonal response, right?

Well, not necessarily.

Understand that pro bodybuilders are essentially walking pharmacies. They take large doses of a variety of anabolic hormones that keep hormone levels sky-high 24/7. The effects of exercise on hormone levels, on the other hand, are transient and last for no more than an hour or two after a workout. The difference between chronically high hormonal levels and a hormonal spike is the difference between apples and tangerines: You just can't compare the two.

There has been extensive research on the so-called "hormone hypothesis" that proposes post-exercise hormonal elevations are primary drivers of muscle growth. Overall, the findings are unconvincing, with most studies failing to support a significant hypertrophic effect of these acute hormonal fluctuations (17). That said, it remains possible that the post-exercise hormone response may play a minor role in anabolic processes, perhaps by increasing the sensitivity of androgen receptors that bind testosterone to facilitate its anabolic actions in the muscle cell (11). Regardless, the body of research indicates that you shouldn't program workouts by attempting to maximize hormonal elevations. Unfortunately, there also is little evidence that resistance training significantly influences chronic hormone levels, so this shouldn't be a programming concern either.

THE MYOKINE FACTOR

While exercise-induced hormonal elevations don't appear to significantly drive anabolism, various intrinsic muscular factors are theorized to be important regulators of growth. These substances, called myokines, are secreted by muscles in response to various stimuli (i.e., mechanical tension, metabolic stress, muscle damage). Each myokine has a somewhat different role in muscle development, carrying out diverse effects on intracellular signaling, satellite cell activity, and other anabolic functions.

As previously mentioned, of the various forms of IGF-1, MGF is considered the most relevant to exercise-induced hypertrophy. Current research indicates that the activation of MGF kickstarts muscle growth in a variety of ways, such as increasing the rate of protein synthesis, activating satellite cells, and increasing muscle calcium levels (3). MGF appears to be especially sensitive to muscle damage, and metabolic stress also may enhance its release.

The interleukins (ILs) represent another important class of myokines. ILs are a family of immuno-inflammatory agents. Several ILs have been identified in muscle tissue, each having distinct roles in its development. Although chronically elevated IL levels are associated with catabolic effects, their acute secretion in response to exercise is believed to enhance muscle size. Research indicates that one myokine in particular, IL-15, is upregulated during resistance training and may play a prominent role in the ensuing growth process (13).

Numerous additional myokines have been implicated in the muscle-building process such as hepato growth factor, fibroblast growth factor, leukemia inhibitory factor, among others. Given their diverse targets, the production of myokines during exercise would seem to have a synergistic effect on growth processes with the extent of their actions adding to the magnitude of gains.

Intriguingly, some myokines have catabolic effects on muscle tissue. For example, a myokine called myostatin is a known negative regulator of muscle development; its release within muscle impairs anabolism and satellite cell function, blunting growth capacity (6). A breed of cattle called the Belgian Blue, which possesses a mutation for the myostatin gene and thus knocks out its ability to produce the myokine, look like they're on a megadose of steroids—so much so they are commonly referred to as "Schwarzenegger cattle." Resistance exercise not only elevates the release of anabolic myokines but also suppresses myostatin production and other catabolic agents to optimize the body's anabolic environment.

FINAL THOUGHTS

The mechanisms of muscle growth are highly complex and involve the intricate signaling of various pathways within the cells. The growth process is supported by satellite cell activity as well as the interaction of various hormones and myokines. Maximizing these factors requires a training routine that optimizes mechanical tension, perhaps in concert with muscle damage and metabolic stress, in a manner that progressively challenges your neuromuscular system to adapt. Chapter 2 details the factors that go into creating such a routine.

M.A.X. PERIODIZATION

Without question, building muscle is the product of consistent, hard training; to make appreciable gains you must regularly push your body beyond its present capacity (an extrapolation of the principle of overload discussed in chapter 1). That said, an often-overlooked factor in achieving a terrific physique is proper planning. An old adage states, "If you fail to plan, you are planning to fail."

With respect to exercise, never was a saying more apt.

Think of it this way: You wouldn't embark on a road trip without first mapping out your destination, right? If you don't plan your route, you're bound to get lost. At best, it'll take you longer to get where you want to go; at worst, you may never get there. Yet, in effect, this is how many people approach their workouts. It's all too common for a person to aimlessly wander around the gym, thinking, "What should I do now?" Such a haphazard approach is doomed to produce substandard results. To maximize your body's genetic potential, you must individualize a plan that is consistent with your training goals. Each workout must fit into the overall scheme of what you are trying to accomplish, and you must properly execute the plan every time you hit the gym.

Central to creating an individualized training plan is the **principle of specificity**. This principle dictates that the results you get from training are specific to the type of exercise program you perform. For example, if you jog for two hours every day, your body will adapt by improving its capacity for aerobic endurance. The quantity of mitochondria in your muscles will increase, as will the activity of various aerobic enzymes. Intense weight training, on the other hand, leads to improved neural responses and increases in the size and force-producing capacity of muscle fibers.

Bottom line: Whatever your fitness goals, your training program must focus on eliciting adaptations that are specific to these goals.

Planning, however, isn't quite as simple as following a cookie-cutter training routine. One of the biggest mistakes a lifter can make is to perform the same exercises in the same fashion over and over. Ultimately the body gets used to the same-old, same-old, which diminishes its drive for further adaptation. What's more, boredom sets in, which in turn brings about a condition called monotonous overtraining that can cause a maladaptation of the neuromuscular system. The upshot: Progress slows to a crawl, inevitably leading to a training plateau or, worse, regression. Only by continuously imposing novel training stimuli in a progressive manner is there an impetus for continued improvement.

A BETTER WAY TO PLAN

How can you structure an exercise program that allows you to make ongoing progress and avoid that dreaded training plateau? The solution can be summed up in one word: **periodization**. Originally developed by Russian strength coaches to prepare their athletes for Olympic competition, periodization refers to the systematic manipulation of the variables of an exercise program (reps, sets, rest intervals, etc.) in a manner that optimizes a given fitness component. In effect, periodization can be thought of as a fancy term for describing an organized system to help guide exercise planning. Here's the scoop.

The traditional periodized program, commonly known as linear periodization, is divided into three components: macrocycle, mesocycle, and microcycle. The macrocycle customarily represents the entire training year but can vary from several months to up to four years. The macrocycle is subdivided into two or more mesocycles that last from several weeks to several months. Mesocycles are subdivided into microcycles of one to four weeks; each microcycle consists of individual training sessions.

An alternative to the traditional periodization model is undulating periodization. Rather than dividing training cycles over months or years, undulating periodization uses a nonlinear approach in which variables are manipulated over short time periods, generally on a week-to-week or even session-to-session basis.

If all this periodization talk sounds a bit fuzzy, don't worry. It will all make sense soon.

The basis of periodization can be traced to the general adaptation syndrome (GAS)—a theory coined in the 1930s by Austrian scientist Hans Selye. During the course of his research, Selye noticed that the body undergoes a triphasic response to stress. First comes the alarm stage, in which the body responds to a new stress by eliciting an acute fight-or-flight response. With repeated exposure to the stressor, the body enters a resistance stage, in which it supercompensates to deal with the stress. If the stressor persists for an extended time, however, the body becomes unable to adapt and enters the exhaustion stage. Ultimately the body's resources become depleted, resulting in an inability to maintain normal bodily function. This leads to a chronic disease state.

Given that exercise is a potent stressor, the GAS theory is relevant to program design. A training cycle should be continued just long enough to elicit an adaptive response (i.e., the upper edge of the resistance stage). Once this critical point is reached, a new stimulus must be applied in order to sustain progress. At various points throughout the cycle, periods of lower-intensity exercise must be interspersed with periods of higher-intensity exercise to avoid entering the exhaustion stage.

That said, it can be beneficial to occasionally push your body to the brink of the exhaustion stage during the course of a periodized routine. Doing so brings about a phenomenon called functional overreaching. Short-term overreaching can optimize the body's ability to supercompensate, thereby maximizing muscle development. The key is to limit overreaching to very brief periods, generally no more than a few weeks, so as to promote positive (functional) adaptations. If overreaching persists for too long, it inevitably leads to a nonfunctional response, potentially devolving into overtraining and a corresponding decrease in results. As an analogy, think of walking to the edge of the cliff to witness a beautiful view of the landscape below. The closer you get to the edge, the better your view. But go too far and you'll suffer serious repercussions. Similarly, you want to take your body to the edge of the cliff from a training standpoint without going over the edge. It's a rather fine line and, when in doubt, you should err on the side of caution.

An important point of note: Periodization is a concept, not a defined way to program. Think of it as a structured method to plan workouts over time. The planning process doesn't have to follow traditional norms, nor does it have to be overly complex. Rather, it must address the ongoing response to training stimuli by adjusting program variables to meet the long-term goals of the individual. The specifics of how to go about planning are part science, part art. Thus, any periodized program—including the one outlined in this book—should not be considered a rigid workout plan, but rather a template that must be customized to your own unique needs and abilities for optimal results.

M.A.X. MUSCLE PLAN:
A PERIODIZED APPROACH

The M.A.X. Muscle Plan is a six-month periodized program designed to maximize your muscular potential. This program can be considered a hybrid of the linear and undulating periodization models. Similar to linear periodization, it includes three mesocycles: a M.A.X. strength phase, a M.A.X. metabolic phase, and a M.A.X. muscle phase. But consistent with undulating periodization, it uses a technique called block periodization in which variables are manipulated on a semiweekly basis. If properly employed, the objective of the plan is to achieve "peak" muscularity at the end of the six-month program. What follows is a discussion of the training variables that will be manipulated over the course of the program.

VOLUME

Research consistently shows that training volume is a primary driver of hypertrophy. Some fitness researchers consider it the most important modifiable variable for exercise-induced muscle growth (5).

Simply stated, volume is the amount of exercise you perform over a given time period (usually expressed on a weekly basis). Volume can be expressed in several ways. **Set volume**, determined by the number of sets performed for a given exercise, is the most common measure of volume, both in research and practice. **Repetition volume**, calculated by adding up the total number of repetitions performed for a given exercise, represents another popular way to express volume. Finally, **volume load**, assessed by multiplying the total number of repetitions by the amount of weight used in an exercise across sets, has been proposed as a superior volume metric. However, although volume load provides a good gauge of total work performed, its relevance to hypertrophy hasn't been well studied and thus its utility remains somewhat questionable in this regard. For our purposes, we'll keep it simple and use set volume for calculation of this variable as this constitutes the majority of research and aligns with the general practice of the bodybuilding community.

Traditional lifting protocols, which date back to the classic DeLorme-Watkins method developed in the late 1940s, advocated performing three sets of each exercise in a workout. For decades thereafter this paradigm was considered standard advice. Beginning in the early 1970s, however, some in the fitness field began to challenge the wisdom of multiple-set training. Arthur Jones, founder of Nautilus, is credited as the first to put forth the notion that only a single set is required to maximally stimulate growth. Jones argued that as long as a set is performed to muscle failure, any additional sets are superfluous and actually may be counterproductive to muscle development. This theory, which came to be known as high-intensity training (HIT), was subsequently embraced by Mike Mentzer, Ellington Darden, and other notables in the industry. Today, HIT (not to be confused with high-intensity interval training—HIIT, as discussed in chapter 12) continues to enjoy a following within a subset of the lifting population.

Does HIT work? Absolutely. Provided that you train sufficiently hard, a HIT routine increases strength and builds muscle. If you're pressed for time, it can be an efficient alternative to multi-set training. I'd go so far as to say that a majority of muscular gains can be achieved with relatively low-volume protocols.

That said, if you want to get the most of your genetic potential, manipulating volume is a key factor for optimizing results. A meta-analysis showed a clear benefit for higher- versus lower-volume protocols, with almost double the percentage of gains seen when performing 10 or more sets per muscle per week compared to less than 5 sets (18). These findings indicate that 10 or more sets per muscle per week is a good starting point when programming volume for hypertrophy-oriented training cycles. Emerging research also shows a fairly large interindividual response to volume, with some responding well to fairly low levels of volume and others requiring substantially higher levels (10); this reinforces the importance of customizing prescription based on response.

The question then becomes: How do you go about determining your own individual training volume? My advice is to begin at the lower end of the range of the guidelines and then adjust the amount of volume accordingly based on your response. Although somewhat speculative, logic dictates that the dose-response relationship between volume and hypertrophy follows an inverted U-shaped (i.e., hormetic) curve, whereby an excessive number of sets would have a detrimental effect on gains. The concept of "trial and error" therefore is an essential process in translating exercise-related research into practical application for each individual.

Moreover, there is a theoretical benefit to performing higher volumes for relatively brief periods of time. The human body is very resilient. It can tolerate, and even thrive, during brief periods of intense stress. However, if the stressor persists over extended periods of time, it ultimately overwhelms the body's adaptive processes, causing an impaired response. Thus, progressively increasing volume from lower (e.g., approximately 10 sets per muscle per week) to higher (e.g., approximately 20 sets per muscle per week) levels over a training cycle may help to promote a state of functional overreaching, which in turn culminates in a peaking of muscle growth while diminishing the potential for overtraining.

Here's another salient point: Overtraining is the product of an excessive accumulation of all the intense exercise you perform for the entire body (see the Understanding Overtraining sidebar in this chapter), not for a given muscle. Thus, think of volume as you would a monetary budget. If you have a fixed amount of money, you can spend up to that limit on virtually anything you desire. However, if you choose to purchase an expensive car that takes up half of your budget, realize that you only have a limited amount of cash left for basic needs such as food and shelter. Your "volume budget" works in a similar manner. Although volume guidelines are based on weekly sets per muscle group, it's misguided to assume that all muscles need the same amount of volume; in actuality, some may benefit more than others. Accordingly, apportion volume based on your individual needs, prioritizing lagging muscles and de-emphasizing muscles that respond well to training. For example, say you have a training cycle that consists of 100 sets per week for all your major muscle groups. Let's also say that you consider your back musculature a lagging area and your chest a strong point. As opposed to performing 15 sets for each of these muscle groups, you instead may choose to allocate 25 sets per week to your back musculature while performing just 5 sets for your chest. A similar approach should be undertaken for all your muscles, prioritizing volume based on their responsiveness. In this way, you make efficient use of your sets while minimizing the potential for overtraining.

It's also important to factor ancillary muscular stimulation into the volume equation. This is particularly true of the limb muscles. The biceps and triceps receive substantial stimulation in multi-joint exercises such as rows, pull-downs, and presses. Similarly, albeit to a lesser extent, the hamstrings and calves are activated in compound lower-body movements such as squats and lunges. In addition, the abdominals receive extensive static work in exercises requiring stabilization of the torso; even muscles such as the sternal and clavicular heads of the pectorals are worked in movements involving shoulder extension (such as the bent row) and shoulder flexion (such as the front raise), respectively.

Although stimulation of ancillary muscles necessarily impacts volume requirements, determining how to take this information into account becomes somewhat problematic because research remains inconclusive on the topic. A simple, logical approach is to consider biceps and triceps work for each multi-joint upper-body exercise as half a set, and hamstrings and calves work for multi-joint lower-body movements as a quarter of a set; the "direct" single-joint work for these muscle groups then can be adjusted based on this formula. With other muscles or portions thereof (posterior delts, upper and lower pecs, etc.), the ancillary stimulation probably is not meaningful enough to be worthy of consideration.

The level of fatigue produced by a given exercise is another issue that needs to be taken into account when programming volume. As a general rule, single-joint exercises are less taxing than multi-joint exercises, and therefore a greater volume can be performed for single-joint movements without eliciting undue systemic fatigue. For example, the standing barbell military press (a compound exercise) generates substantially more neuromuscular fatigue compared to a dumbbell lateral raise; accordingly, you can handle more volume for the lateral raise without overtaxing the body. Similarly, machine-based exercises tend to be less fatiguing than free weight movements, thereby allowing greater volumes when using machines.

The M.A.X. Muscle Plan periodizes volume in a systematic fashion, progressing from cycles of lower volume to those with higher volume. This is particularly evident in the M.A.X. muscle phase, where each block progressively increases volume to culminate in an "overreaching" block designed to bring about hypertrophic supercompensation. Provided you manage volume based on your individual response as described above, the graded stress to your neuromuscular system over the course of this phase should help achieve peak muscle development upon its completion.

FREQUENCY

Frequency of training can be looked at in two ways. First, it can refer to the number of exercise sessions you perform in a given period of time, usually reported on a weekly basis. The second way, which is perhaps of more relevance to hypertrophy programs, refers to how frequently a given muscle group is worked—again, generally calculated per week. In actuality, the two are somewhat interrelated.

Research seems to show fairly similar muscle growth irrespective of how many times a muscle group is trained (20). A slight hypertrophic advantage seems to exist for training a muscle twice per week compared to once, but the overall difference is fairly modest and thus of questionable practical significance. Moreover, no additional benefits are seen for training a muscle more than twice weekly.

There's a caveat to these findings, however: They are specific to routines where volume is equated between muscle groups.

Evidence indicates there is in fact a benefit to greater weekly per-muscle frequencies when volume is not equated (20), particularly with the performance of higher training volumes. While a hard cutoff can't be established, it appears that when volume exceeds approximately 10 sets per muscle in a session, it's best to split that volume over multiple days. For example, say your routine consists of 20 weekly sets for the quads. Rather than performing all these sets in a single workout, it's better to split up the volume into two sessions of 10 sets per week. If the routine involves 30 weekly sets for a given muscle group, three weekly sessions of 10 sets would be preferable.

Although the reason for the volume–frequency relationship isn't completely clear, it may be that there's an upper limit to the amount of muscle proteins that the body can synthesize from a given training session. Recall that hypertrophy is predicated on muscle protein balance; to build muscle, synthesis of new proteins must exceed breakdown over time. If muscle protein synthesis reaches a threshold at a certain amount of volume (e.g., 10 sets), any additional sets in essence will be "wasted" from a muscle-building standpoint. Spreading out the volume over the course of the week therefore would allow for greater weekly protein synthesis, conceivably enhancing long-term muscle growth.

It also should be noted that long training bouts tend to be associated with a reduced intensity of effort, decreased motivation, and alterations in immune response. Think about it logically. Your ability to train hard is optimal early in a training session when you are fresh. As the session wears on, your energy and focus gradually wane, reducing the quality of the sets performed later in the workout. Thus, it's generally best to limit intensive workouts to no more than 60-90 minutes in length to ensure maximal training capacity throughout each lifting session. When weekly volume levels are high, you'll therefore need to increase the frequency of training to stay within this prescribed workout duration.

Hence, consider frequency as a tool that can and should be manipulated to accommodate weekly per-muscle training volume. As a general rule, at least three weekly resistance training sessions are necessary to maximize muscle development; you simply cannot accumulate sufficient volume for all your body's muscle groups training one or two days per week. That said, a greater frequency can potentially augment results when performing higher volumes. Specifically, if the volume for a given muscle group is relatively high, distribute it across additional weekly workouts so that a single session does not exceed approximately 10 sets for that muscle group.

Some fitness pros have proposed that you should distribute volume over six or seven days a week so that muscles are worked in each session with a fewer number of sets per workout. In support for this hypothesis, proponents point to a study carried out at the Norwegian School of Sport Sciences, which has come to be known as the "Norwegian Frequency Project." The study randomized members of the Norwegian powerlifting team to perform either four sets per exercise on three nonconsecutive days per week or two sets per exercise on six consecutive days. After 16 weeks, only the daily training group showed increases in muscle size; the group training three days per week had no gains!

On the surface, the findings appear compelling. But before jumping on the high-frequency bandwagon, consider a few things. First and foremost, the results of this study were presented as a conference abstract in 2012; at the time of publication of this book, the study still had yet to be published in a peer-reviewed journal. Thus, it is impossible to scrutinize the study's methodology and determine what, if any, issues may have influenced results. That said, I had the opportunity to speak to one of the lead researchers who informed me that the protocol was designed as a powerlifting study, not a bodybuilding study. The exercises were limited to the typical "big three" powerlifting movements (squat, deadlift, and bench press), with performance of each set stopped well short of failure. Moreover, the researcher stated that while this was the type of program commonly used for strength development among Norwegian powerlifters, their hypertrophy routines involved reduced frequencies per muscle group with higher training volumes—more typical of bodybuilding-type programs. Of note, two more recent studies with similar designs showed no hypertrophic benefit to very high-frequency training, and there was even some evidence of a detrimental effect (4, 14).

A logical case can be made for allowing a minimum of 48 hours between sessions that target the prime movers in a muscle group because this is the approximate time course of muscle protein synthesis. Theoretically, training a muscle group before protein synthesis has completed its course would cause you to miss out on additional gains for that muscle group, while at the same time resulting in a lost opportunity to potentially enhance gains in other muscle groups. This also goes for secondary synergists. Exercises such as pull-downs and rows require substantial muscle contribution from the elbow flexors (biceps brachii), and pressing movements involve a significant contribution from the elbow extensors (triceps brachii). The greater the involvement of a given synergist during exercise performance, the greater the need for post-exercise recovery.

The fatigue factor also must be taken into account. Not only are the working muscles highly stressed during intense training, but the supporting connective tissues are as well. Shortchanging the recovery process for these tissues impairs future performance, reducing your ability to train at a high level—and it should go without saying that you can't maximize gains if your training capacity is compromised.

That said, as with virtually all applied topics, there are exceptions to every rule. Lagging muscles may benefit from greater volumes, and it sometimes can be beneficial to train them more than three times per week to accommodate the increased volume. This necessarily mandates working that muscle group on back-to-back days. Don't worry; provided the time course of such a cycle is relatively short term (a few weeks), this won't be an issue. As mentioned, the human body is very resilient and can thrive during brief periods of high stress; the key is to effectively manage walking the stress tightrope by not pushing too hard for too long.

Bottom line: Structure your routines to provide adequate recovery time to all muscles receiving significant work in a session.

To an extent, per-muscle training frequency is limited by how you organize your routine. Specifically, you can train either in a total-body fashion in which you work all the major muscles in a single session or by various types of split routines in which you perform multiple exercises for a given number of muscle groups in a session. A benefit of total-body training is that each muscle typically is trained with a greater frequency than in split routines. This is particularly advantageous when the goal is to enhance strength adaptations in multi-joint free weight exercises because motor learning benefits for complex movements are observed with more frequent practice (9).

Total-body routines can be effective for hypertrophy-oriented programs when volume is relatively low. However, body part splits tend to be a better option with the use of higher volumes. Compared with full-body routines, a split routine allows you to better distribute total weekly training volume while affording greater recovery between sessions. From a mechanistic standpoint, this may enable you to use heavier daily training loads and thus generate greater mechanical tension, as well as potentially increase metabolic stress by prolonging the training stimulus within a given muscle group. Importantly, there is no "best" body part split; numerous options exist, and all of them can be viable. The ideal split ultimately will depend on what you are trying to accomplish in a given training cycle specific to your individual needs and abilities.

The M.A.X. Muscle Plan varies training frequency to best distribute the amount of volume in a given cycle. In most cases, training is carried out either three or four days a week. However, a six-day-a-week cycle is employed in the final block of the muscle phase whereby volume is increased to high levels in an effort to bring about a supercompensatory response. Both total-body and split-body routines are employed to effectively manage the distribution of volume across each training block and phase.

UNDERSTANDING OVERTRAINING

Overtraining, often referred to as overtraining syndrome (OTS), is an exercise-related affliction that affects a sizable number of people who exercise on a regular basis. Because people lack understanding of the subject, it often ends up going undiagnosed.

Simply stated, overtraining results from performing too much strenuous physical activity. However, the exact threshold for overtraining varies from person to person. Some people can tolerate high training volumes and intensities whereas others begin to develop symptoms of overtraining from doing much less. What's more, factors such as nutrition status, sleeping patterns, hormone concentrations, muscle fiber composition, and previous training experience all affect recuperative capacity and, therefore, the point at which overtraining rears its ugly head.

OTS manifests in a systemic manner, affecting multiple bodily processes. In almost all cases, it causes the body to enter a catabolic state. Catabolism is mediated by an increased production of cortisol—a stress hormone secreted by the adrenal cortex—which exerts its influence at the cellular level, impeding muscular repair and function. Making matters worse, a corresponding decrease often occurs in anabolic hormone production (e.g., testosterone, IGF-1). Together, these factors combine to inhibit protein synthesis and accelerate proteolysis (protein breakdown).

In addition, because of a depletion of glutamine stores, OTS suppresses the body's immune system (25). Glutamine is the major source of energy for immune cells, and a steady supply of glutamine is necessary for their proper function. However, glutamine levels are rapidly exhausted when exercise volume is excessively high. Without an adequate amount of this nutrient, the immune system loses its ability to produce antibodies such as lymphocytes, leukocytes, and cytokines. Ultimately, the body's capacity to fight viral and bacterial infections becomes impaired, leading to an increased incidence of illness.

Here are some of the symptoms related to overtraining. If you experience several of these symptoms, you very well might be overtrained. If symptoms persist, get plenty of sleep and don't resume training until you feel mentally and physically ready.

- Increased resting heart rate
- Increased resting blood pressure
- Decreased exercise performance
- Decreased appetite
- Decreased desire to work out
- Increased incidence of injuries
- Increased incidence of infections and flu-like symptoms
- Increased irritability and depression

Some fitness pros have furthered the concept of "localized overtraining," whereby detrimental effects are specific to excessive training of a given muscle or muscle group without affecting other body systems. Localized overtraining is purported to occur when the same muscle group is trained too frequently, with too much volume or too intensely in a given time span. However, such a phenomenon has not been documented in the literature and thus remains speculative.

Without question, there is a diminished benefit from higher training volumes. Once a given muscle has reached its volume limit, additional sets will be of no further benefit for that muscle. Moreover, excessive training of a muscle group, particularly with heavier loads, will overstress joints in a manner that ultimately hastens the onset of soft tissue injuries. Nagging injuries such as lateral epicondylitis (tennis elbow) and patellofemoral pain syndrome (runner's knee) are commonly associated with excessive training focused on a given area of the body. However, the concept of localized overtraining technically doesn't meet the criteria for classification as OTS and can more accurately be called "overuse."

LOAD

Training load dictates the number of repetitions that you can perform for a particular exercise. This is commonly called the repetition range, or rep range. Rep ranges can be classified into three broad categories: low (1-5 reps), moderate (6-12 reps), and high (15 or more reps). Each of these rep ranges involves the use of different energy systems and taxes the neuromuscular system in different ways.

A compelling body of research shows that training in a low rep range is best for increasing muscle strength (17). This should make intuitive sense, given that strength is defined as the ability to exert maximal force. Although gains in muscle mass certainly heighten the ability to produce force, the relationship is not linear because strength gains have a substantial neurological component. Only by lifting heavy can you optimize these neural improvements, which are essential to maximizing absolute strength.

Low-rep, heavy-load sets necessarily involve high levels of mechanical tension. The imposed mechanical stress is high from the outset of a set, resulting in substantial recruitment and stimulation throughout. Because the duration of low-rep sets is relatively brief, energy is primarily derived from the phosphagen system (a.k.a. ATP-creatine phosphate system), with limited contribution from anaerobic glycolysis; thus, metabolic stress is low during this type of training.

At the other end of the loading zone spectrum, a high-rep range is believed to promote adaptations specific to local muscular endurance (i.e., the ability to lift submaximal weights multiple times). Higher-rep sets require substantial contribution from the anaerobic glycolytic energy system to fuel performance. Hence, this training scheme produces substantial metabolic stress. Alternatively, since the load is relatively light, mechanical tension remains relatively low during the initial reps of a set and only increases as you approach fatigue.

A moderate rep range, corresponding to 6-12 reps per set, is a bit of a compromise between heavy- and light-load training. Mechanical tension is generally high throughout a moderate-rep set, although initially not quite as high as when using heavy loads. And because moderate-rep training taps into the anaerobic glycolytic system for energy production, there is substantial metabolite buildup—although less so than during the performance of light-load sets.

For many years, both bodybuilders and exercise scientists alike championed the claim that a moderate rep range was optimal for gains in muscle size. From a research standpoint, this theory was largely predicated on acute studies showing a spike in anabolic hormone production following moderate-rep sets. However, as noted in chapter 1, emerging evidence calls into question the so-called "hormone hypothesis," and the general consensus indicates that transient post-exercise hormonal elevations are of relatively minor consequence to muscular gains (15).

In truth, there is no ideal "hypertrophy range" for repetitions. Research on the topic is now compelling: Similar gains in muscle size can be achieved over a wide spectrum of loading zones (17). But even though you can build appreciable muscle with heavy and light loads, there are some benefits to focusing on moderate loads during a hypertrophy-oriented training cycle. For one, heavy-load training requires the performance of a greater number of sets to achieve comparable muscle growth than when using moderate loads; thus, the use of moderate loads provides a more efficient way to train. Moreover, the combination of heavy loads and high training volumes is a recipe for overtraining and injury, making moderate loads a safer choice for muscle-building goals. Furthermore, the duration of high-rep sets is substantially longer than that of moderate-rep sets. The extended time under tension is accompanied by high levels of metabolic acidosis, causing prolonged discomfort as fatigue ensues. The upshot is that training with high reps to fatigue is not all that enjoyable of an experience; it can be tolerated for short cycles, but most lifters much prefer the use of moderate-rep sets.

All that said, there is good reason to vary rep ranges over the course of a training cycle. Since low-rep training maximizes strength, its inclusion in a hypertrophy-oriented routine can facilitate the use of heavier loads during moderate-rep sets; the corresponding increased mechanical tension achieved conceivably drives a greater growth response. Alternatively, high-rep sets help to improve muscle-buffering capacity, delaying the exercise-induced buildup of lactic acid and thus extending the length of the set. This can transfer to an enhanced ability to pump out additional reps during moderate-rep sets, which in turn enhances the hypertrophic stimulus.

There's another potential benefit to combining rep ranges. Namely, research suggests that people respond differently to different magnitudes of loading

(21); some seem to achieve greater gains with heavier loads while others appear to respond better to using lighter weights. These results may vary between muscle groups. Although speculative, it's conceivable that combining rep ranges might have synergistic effects on hypertrophy, perhaps by targeting different intracellular signaling pathways and thus promoting synergistic effects on muscle protein synthesis. Much still needs to be determined in this regard, but the strategy of varying rep ranges seemingly provides a good cost–benefit ratio. The key is to effectively manage prescription of this variable to promote a safe and productive training environment.

The M.A.X. Muscle Plan incorporates training cycles specific to the three distinct loading zones in a periodized fashion. Moreover, it does so in a manner whereby each loading cycle potentiates the effects of the hypertrophy

CAN YOU TRAIN MUSCLES BASED ON THEIR FIBER TYPE?

Muscle fibers can be classified into two primary types: slow twitch (type I) and fast twitch (type II). Slow-twitch fibers are endurance-oriented fibers that can withstand repeated contractions but have a limited ability to generate force. Fast-twitch fibers, on the other hand, have a substantial capacity for generating force but tend to fatigue easily.

As you probably expect from these descriptions, fast-twitch fibers have a significantly greater capacity for growth than slow-twitch fibers—about 50 percent greater by most accounts (1). Some lifters mistakenly take this to mean that slow-twitch fibers don't get bigger. Not true. Although slow-twitch fibers aren't as responsive to growth as fast-twitch fibers, they nevertheless do hypertrophy when subjected to an overload stimulus. Given that the majority of whole muscles have a significant number of slow-twitch fibers, regardless of individual variance, this can potentially help to maximize whole-muscle girth.

Interestingly, studies show that bodybuilders display greater hypertrophy of slow-twitch fibers than powerlifters. It's hypothesized that this may be due to differences in training methodology—bodybuilders train with higher reps than powerlifters—and seems to explain, at least in part, why bodybuilders are more muscular than powerlifters (although correlation cannot necessarily be taken as causation). In particular, some have speculated that the moderate- to high-rep protocols employed by bodybuilders preferentially target slow-twitch fibers. To date, research remains equivocal on the topic, with some studies showing preferential slow-twitch growth with higher- versus lower-rep training and others failing to observe differences between rep ranges (8). Given the uncertainty of research, it makes sense to cover all bases and train through a spectrum of loading ranges; it may help to enhance the growth response and won't hurt your efforts.

phase, ultimately maximizing muscular gains. You'll start with a strength phase using low reps that involve high levels of mechanical tension; this will enhance your ability to handle heavier loads. You'll then move to a high-rep metabolic phase designed to improve buffering of lactic acid, facilitating your ability to perform more reps at a given submaximal workload. You'll finish the cycle with a muscle phase employing moderate loads designed to provide relatively high levels of mechanical tension while allowing completion of a sufficient volume of training in a time-efficient manner.

The program also makes use of a technique called step loading in which progressive increases in the magnitude of load are followed by a brief deload period within a given training cycle. This structure creates a wavelike loading pattern that allows the use of a broad spectrum of reps within a target rep range while reducing the potential for overtraining. You'll see how this plays out in the training chapters.

REST INTERVAL

The amount of time you take from the end of one set to the beginning of the next is called the rest interval. Rest intervals can be classified into three broad categories: short (approximately 30 seconds or less), moderate (about one to two minutes), and long (approximately three minutes or more).

Until recently, research-based guidelines indicated that hypertrophy training should involve resting at the lower end of the moderate range (approximately one minute between sets). This conclusion was largely based on studies showing greater post-exercise anabolic hormone elevations when limiting rest periods. However, as discussed in chapter 1, acute exercise-induced hormonal elevations don't seem to play much of a role in muscle growth. In fact, emerging evidence suggests that resting at the upper end of the moderate range may be more conducive to muscular gains in trained lifters (7), conceivably because the shorter rest periods compromise the number of reps you're able to perform on succeeding sets. However, the reduction in reps from the use of shorter rest intervals is mainly seen in the performance of compound exercises; single-joint movements tend to show minimal differences in volume load across multiple sets regardless of rest interval duration (23). The practical takeaway from a hypertrophy standpoint is that it makes sense to employ approximately two-minute rest intervals for compound exercises to maintain volume load across sets. Alternatively, resting approximately 60-90 seconds can be employed for single-joint movements because this heightens metabolic stress and thus potentially augments the anabolic response without impacting volume load; at the very least, it serves to make workout sessions more time efficient.

Both longer and shorter rest intervals have their place in a hypertrophy-focused training program. Long rest intervals allow for complete muscular recovery after performance of a set. You need approximately three minutes between sets to fully regain your strength on a given exercise. Full recovery allows you to train with your heaviest weight within a given rep range, ensuring that you generate maximal muscle tension during the ensuing set. This level of recovery is good for increasing both strength and size. On the other hand, any metabolite buildup that may arise dissipates over the course of the rest period, which is good for strength but may reduce a potential avenue for increases in muscle size.

Bottom line: Longer rest intervals are beneficial when your goal is to enhance basic strength.

Short rest intervals basically have the opposite effect. Metabolite accumulation skyrockets with limited rest periods. This not only enhances the body's anabolic environment but also makes your muscles more impervious to lactic acid buildup—factors conceivably beneficial for both muscular endurance and size. The downside is that short rest intervals do not allow sufficient time to fully regain your strength. In fact, strength decrements of up to 50 percent are seen in subsequent sets when rest intervals are limited to 30 seconds. The upshot is that volume load is compromised, reducing muscle-building capacity. Hence, short rest periods are best employed during metabolic cycles intended to enhance muscle-buffering capacity.

The M.A.X. Muscle Plan varies rest periods depending on both the goal of the mesocycle as well as the specific qualities of the exercise performed. Long rest intervals are performed during the strength phase to provide full recuperation of maximal strength capacity. Alternatively, short rest periods are employed in the metabolic phase so as to heighten metabolite buildup and enhance local muscle endurance-oriented adaptations. During the muscle phase, rest periods vary between one to two minutes, with longer intervals used in the compound exercises and shorter intervals employed for single-joint movements.

EFFORT

The effort you expend during a set will significantly affect your results. Muscular gains are achieved only by challenging your muscles beyond their present capacity. This is a basic application of the principle of overload, as discussed in chapter 1. If you don't continually challenge your muscles, they have no impetus to grow. Period.

One of the most controversial topics among fitness professionals is whether a benefit exists for training to momentary muscle failure, the point during a set at which muscles can no longer produce enough force to complete the lift. In one camp are those who claim you should reach failure on every set of every exercise. In another camp are those who say failure is unnecessary and even counterproductive to results. Who's right? If the goal is muscle development, the answer seems to lie somewhere between these two extremes.

Current research fails to show superiority of failure training for hypertrophy when compared to stopping a rep or two short of failure; with respect to strength, there appears to be a slight negative effect of going to failure. However, a couple of important caveats must be considered in this regard. For one, all studies to date have investigated training to failure versus not training to failure for every set in the research protocol. However, the decision to employ failure training doesn't necessarily have to be an either-or choice. There is no research investigating the use of failure training on a limited number of sets—say the last set or two of a given exercise. Moreover, although several studies on the topic have employed "resistance-trained" individuals, none of the participants on average can be considered highly trained. It is conceivable that those with considerable training experience, particularly competitive physique athletes, require a very high level of stimulus to promote additional growth and hence may benefit from selective incorporation of failure training.

A perceived benefit of training to failure is that it can increase stimulation of muscle fibers. When a lifter becomes fatigued, a progressively greater number of fibers are recruited to continue muscular activity. Moreover, the spectrum of fibers is kept under tension at high firing rates, conceivably providing an additional stimulus for growth.

When moderate to high reps are used, training to failure also may enhance exercise-induced metabolic stress. You don't have to be an exercise scientist to know that you get a greater pump—which is indicative of a high degree of cell swelling—when you go all out in a set. Test-tube research shows these acute effects are associated with greater protein synthesis, which potentially may lead to increased long-term muscle growth.

On the other hand, training to failure has a potential downside. At the very least, failure training increases the time needed to recover between sets. Longer rest intervals are therefore needed to preserve volume load, which negatively affects the time efficiency of your workout. Moreover, consistently pushing to fatigue on a weekly basis increases the potential for overtraining and psychological burnout. Negative alterations in resting hormone concentrations—a widely used marker of overtraining—have been reported when lifters repeatedly trained to failure over time (12). Thus, although some failure training may help to maximize muscle development, pushing too hard too often is almost certainly destined to have a negative effect.

How much is too much? Tough to say. Some lifters can tolerate failure training more readily than others. The key is to periodize this variable over the course of a training cycle. If any initial signs of overtraining manifest, reduce the frequency of sets performed to failure accordingly.

How do you quantify effort if you don't train to failure? A simple method is to use a concept called **repetitions in reserve** (RIR). Simply stated, RIR measures your perceived proximity to failure. An RIR of "0" means you have reached muscle failure; an RIR of "1" indicates you had one rep left in the tank; an RIR of "2" indicates you were two reps short of failure, and so on. For example, if you perform a 10-rep set at an RIR of 2, this indicates you could have done 12 reps at that given load. The RIR scale has been validated

Table 2.1   Repetitions in Reserve Scale

RIR	INTENSITY OF EFFORT
0	Maximum effort
0.5	Perhaps could have done 1 more repetition
1	Definitely could have done 1 more repetition
1.5	Could have done 1 more repetition, perhaps even 2
2	Definitely could have done 2 more repetitions
2.5	Could have done 2 more repetitions, perhaps even 3
3	Definitely could have done 3 more repetitions
3.5	Could have done 3 more repetitions, perhaps even 4
4	Definitely could have done 4 more repetitions
4.5	Could have done 4 more repetitions, perhaps even 5
≥5	Definitely could have done 5 or more repetitions

Adapted from E.R. Helms, J. Cronin, A. Storey, and M.C. Zourdos, "Application of the Repetitions in Reserve-Based Rating of Perceived Exertion Scale for Resistance Training," *Strength and Conditioning Journal* 38, no. 4 (2016): 42-49. (11)

by research (13); accuracy tends to improve the more you use the scale. See table 2.1 for an RIR scale you can use to gauge effort during resistance training.

The M.A.X. Muscle Plan judiciously incorporates failure training across the program. The RIR concept is employed to help guide your level of effort from set to set. The majority of working sets will be carried out short of failure, using an RIR of 1 to 3. However, you will selectively go all out throughout portions of each cycle, generally reserving such efforts for the last set of an exercise.

TEMPO

Tempo refers to the speed with which you perform a repetition. It is specific to the three types of contractions: concentric, eccentric, and isometric. The concentric, or positive, portion of a rep occurs when you lift a weight against the force of gravity; the eccentric, or negative, portion of a rep occurs when you lower a weight in the direction of gravity; and the isometric, or static, portion of a rep occurs when the weight is being held statically while producing force. For example, the concentric portion of a biceps curl takes place when you bring the dumbbell up toward your shoulders. Alternatively, lowering the dumbbell constitutes the eccentric phase of the lift. The isometric phase occurs at the top position and bottom position of the lift because the weight is stationary at these points.

Tempo can be expressed as a four-digit number separated by hyphens in which the first number represents the concentric phase, the second number the isometric phase at the top of the lift, the third number the eccentric phase, and the fourth number the isometric phase at the bottom of the lift. In the example of the biceps curl, a tempo of 1-0-3-0 means that the concentric phase lasts one second, the isometric phase at the top of the lift is imperceptible, the eccentric phase lasts three seconds, and the isometric phase at the bottom of the lift is imperceptible.

Research shows little difference in muscle growth between faster (1-0-1-0) compared with slower (3-0-3-0) tempos (16). However, both science and in-the-trenches experience suggest that rather than gauging tempo based on the actual speed of repetition, it's more relevant to focus on the quality of the muscular contraction. This is best accomplished by employing a concept called the **mind–muscle connection** (a.k.a. an internal focus of attention) whereby you consciously focus on making the target muscle work throughout each rep. For example, during performance of the bent barbell row, focus on actively engaging the lats as you pull the weight toward your torso. Then focus on allowing the lats to stretch as you lower the weight back to the start position. The process repeats for each repetition, always keeping the target muscle engaged throughout the entire set.

All too often, lifters direct their efforts to the concentric action, neglecting the eccentric phase of movement. Big mistake. Research shows that eccentric actions are just as important, if not more so, for promoting hypertrophy (19). Here's why. Eccentric actions involve lengthening a muscle under tension, which results in a preferential recruitment of fast-twitch fibers. Because fewer fibers are called on to produce force during eccentric movement, those that are active are forced to bear a greater amount of tension. As a result, microtrauma is increased, leading to greater remodeling of the working fibers, particularly those at the insertion (distal portion) of the muscle. In fact, there is evidence that eccentric and concentric actions are synergistic, promoting more complete muscle development than either action alone (6). The only way to get the full benefit from training eccentrically is by lowering weights under control; simply allowing gravity to take over causes you to miss out on valuable gains. Again, you don't need to adhere to a specific tempo; maintaining a mind–muscle connection during the eccentric phase will effectively ensure that the target muscle is kept under sufficient tension.

It's worth noting that the isometric portion of the lift is less of a concern from a muscle-development standpoint. Some fitness pros recommend holding the top phase of the lift for a second or so to generate a peak muscular contraction. Research to support such a practice, however, is lacking. Your best bet is to maintain constant tension on the target muscle by not locking out the joint at the top of the lift. Provided that you perform each rep in a smooth, controlled fashion with a strong mind–muscle connection, eliciting a peak isometric contraction seems to be superfluous.

I'll note that the beneficial effects of a mind–muscle connection are specific to hypertrophy-oriented training. If the goal is to maximize strength, it is preferable to employ an external focus of attention whereby you think about the outcome of the movement. For example, in the bench press exercise, an external focus cue could be to "push the bar through the ceiling." This

SUPERSLOW TRAINING

The technique of superslow training has gained a modicum of popularity over the years. In this form of resistance exercise training, each repetition takes about 15 seconds to complete (e.g., 10-0-5-0). It's based on the concept that performing repetitions at an extremely slow tempo reduces momentum and therefore increases the forces on the target muscle. In addition, by reducing momentum, the potential for injury is supposedly decreased. Although this may sound logical, closer scrutiny suggests otherwise.

First, the effects of momentum on training are wildly overstated. Provided that weights are lifted in a controlled fashion, the target muscles perform the majority of the work; momentum is not a determining factor. What's more, simply slowing the speed of repetitions has no apparent effect on reducing injuries. In fact, the injury rate for those who train with proper form and technique in a traditional protocol is extremely low. Thus, the underlying science behind the superslow claims simply doesn't add up.

In addition to being extremely tedious for most lifters, superslow training is suboptimal from a muscle-building standpoint. Although direct research on the topic is limited, the few studies that have been carried out show an advantage to more traditional tempo protocols (3, 22). At the very least, there is no evidence of an inherent advantage to training in superslow fashion, and it is quite possibly a detriment to the practice, making it a poor cost–benefit strategy.

is consistent with the constrained-action hypothesis, which proposes that focusing externally facilitates more effective and efficient movement patterns (26), thereby enhancing performance during outcome-oriented tasks such as those involving heavy lifting.

The M.A.X. Muscle Plan incorporates an external attentional focus during the strength phase, where you concentrate on moving the weight as explosively as possible. Alternatively, during the metabolic and muscle phases, you'll employ a mind–muscle connection throughout each lift. The focus here will be to visualize the working muscle(s) and force them to remain active on both the concentric and eccentric portions of every repetition.

EXERCISE SELECTION

Exercise selection refers to the assortment of exercises you perform throughout a training routine. Varying exercise selection is beneficial to muscle development for several reasons. First, muscles often have different attachment sites (where muscles attach to bone). Depending on the exercise performed, the point of attachment may increase leverage in one aspect of the muscle while decreasing leverage in another aspect. For example, the trapezius (a large muscle in the back) is subdivided so that the upper aspect elevates the scapula, the middle aspect abducts the scapula, and the lower portion depresses the scapula. Hence, shrugs primarily work the upper traps, rows the middle traps, and lat pull-downs the lower traps. Other muscles such as the pectoralis major (the primary chest muscle), deltoids, and triceps are segmented into distinct heads, and each head is responsible for carrying out different joint actions. Thus, an assortment of exercises ensures complete stimulation of all fibers.

Additionally, muscle fibers don't necessarily span the entire length of the muscle as commonly believed. The rectus abdominis, for example, is subdivided by several fibrous bands called tendinous inscriptions (the connective tissue that gives the abs their six-pack appearance), and the upper and lower segments are supplied by different nerve branches. Other muscles such as the sartorius, gracilis, and various aspects of the hamstrings are similarly subdivided by one or more fibrous bands and innervated by separate nerves. These architectural differences allow you to selectively target portions of a muscle by performing specific movements.

Bottom line: No single exercise can effectively maximize development of a muscle group. You can achieve full development only by varying exercise selection so that muscles are worked from different angles in all planes of movement. Even changing hand spacing or foot stance in a movement can bring about distinct muscular adaptations, thus improving symmetry and development.

Exercises can be classified into two broad categories: multi-joint and single joint. Multi-joint (a.k.a. compound) exercises require two or more joints to carry out the movement. An example is the bench press, in which the shoulder and elbow joints are both involved to lift the weight. Single-joint exercises require movement of only one joint to complete a repetition. An example is the biceps curl, in which the elbow joint is solely responsible for lifting the weight. Both single- and multi-joint exercises have a place in a muscle-building routine.

How often should you change exercises? To an extent, this depends on the phase of the periodization cycle. Strength improvements tend to be maximized with a limited number of exercises because maximal strength is highly dependent on neuromuscular factors involving the connection between the brain, nervous system, and muscles. The goal is to hardwire the movements into your neural circuitry. The more frequently you perform a given exercise, the more your body develops an affinity for the movement.

During a hypertrophy cycle, on the other hand, a more frequent rotation of exercises is desirable. The goal is to vary parameters such as angle of pull, exercise modality, and so on to elicit different activation patterns within whole muscles and muscle compartments and to provide a unique stimulus to muscle fibers that heightens microtrauma. That said, too much variation can have a negative effect on exercise performance, thereby impairing the amount of load that can be handled and, consequently, diminishing mechanical tension. This is primarily specific to more complex exercises, particularly free weight, multi-joint movements such as squats, rows, and presses performed with barbells and dumbbells. The need for coordination is high in these movements, requiring fairly regular practice to maintain proficiency in performance. On the other hand, single-joint exercises and machine-based movements require less skill to carry out. You can take several months off from performing a biceps curl or leg extension and have little to no drop off in performance when returning to perform the movement. Therefore, a good rule of thumb is to keep the more complex exercises as staples in your regular routine while more frequently rotating performance of those that require less skill to complete.

The M.A.X. Muscle Plan structures exercise selection based on the goals of the mesocycle. Both the strength and metabolic phases keep exercises fairly constant throughout each cycle. There is a focus on compound movements in these phases, with limited variation. On the other hand, the muscle phase emphasizes working muscles from different planes and angles with a greater variety of movements. Complex exercises, particularly those involving free

UNSTABLE SURFACES

Wobble boards, Swiss balls, DynaDiscs, BOSU, and other unstable-surface devices are popular pieces of gym equipment often associated with the concept of "functional training." Some proponents have gone as far as to claim that every exercise should be performed on an unstable surface to optimize functional capacity. Although these implements can help you attain certain fitness goals, their use is generally not warranted in a muscle-building routine.

From a muscle-building standpoint, the perceived benefit of unstable-surface training is actually its biggest weakness. Lifting weights on an unstable surface requires extensive activation of the core musculature. More core activation may sound like a good thing, but when you consider the trade-off, it's not. The increased involvement of the muscles of the abs and lower back comes at the expense of the prime movers (agonists)—you simply can't lift as much weight when training on an unstable surface. Studies show that force output is as much as 70 percent lower when performing exercises on an unstable surface than when performing exercises on a stable surface (2). Such large reductions in force output diminish dynamic tension to the target muscles, impairing hypertrophic adaptations.

There is an exception: The use of unstable surfaces in exercises that directly work the core musculature can be beneficial in a hypertrophy-oriented routine. This makes sense because unstable surfaces increase core activation. The abs in particular may benefit from unstable-surface training. Research shows that crunches performed on a Swiss ball elicit significantly greater muscle activity in the upper and lower rectus abdominis and the external obliques than crunches performed under stable conditions (24). Thus, adding in some unstable-surface exercises for direct ab work can potentially enhance muscle development of the midsection.

weights and multiple joints, are held constant throughout the mesocycle while simpler movements are rotated more frequently.

GETTING STARTED

You now have all the background necessary to begin the M.A.X. Muscle Plan. The program is designed to take all the guesswork out of training. I provide a structured template to follow, with sample routines for every week of each phase of the program. Exercises, sets, reps, and rest intervals are listed in chart form for easy reference. All you have to do is put in the dedication and effort.

Note that the sample routines are general blueprints for structuring your routine. Consistent with the **principle of individuality**, you can and should adjust exercise variables to best suit your genetic makeup, psychological stresses, age, training experience, health status, and recovery rate. The best advice I can give is to remain in tune with your body and be willing to experiment based on your individual response. Ultimately, everyone becomes their own n = 1 study.

Also note that the exercises provided in the routines are merely suggestions. If a certain movement doesn't feel right to you or if you don't have access to a particular piece of equipment, then simply substitute a different exercise. Just make sure the replacement is comparable to the one listed and targets similar muscles in the same plane of movement. Say, for example, that a particular routine calls for a barbell bench press, but you don't have access to an Olympic bar or the necessary number of plates. No problem. Perform a dumbbell bench press instead. Although the two exercises are not identical, they work essentially the same muscles in similar ways.

Finally, I highly recommend that you maintain a training diary over the course of this program. Write down every rep of every set of every exercise for every workout. Moreover, make notes of any lifestyle factors that may be relevant such as how you felt during a given training session, whether you slept well the previous night, what you ate and drank that day, and so on; as a general rule, the more info, the better. Charting each workout in this fashion gives you an objective gauge of your progress over time. It's hard data that isn't prone to memory lapse, as opposed to trying to recall what you did retrospectively. This can prove invaluable when attempting to determine what's working and what isn't.

Review your diary on a semiregular basis. Look for patterns that may reveal why you performed well or not over a given time period. Assess whether anything could be tweaked for better results. Then use what you learned about the science of muscle development in combination with your personal experience to decide on the best strategy for improvement going forward. Just make sure you take emotion out of the equation and remain as objective as possible in your assessment; it's key to optimizing results.

By now you're undoubtedly stoked to begin the routine, so if you're ready and willing to take your physique to the next level, read on.

EXERCISES FOR THE BACK, CHEST, AND ABDOMEN

This chapter describes and illustrates exercises for the chest, back, and abdominal muscles. The back and chest are made up of the most powerful muscles in the upper body. Development of this musculature will ultimately delineate the shape of your physique and enhance your ability to carry out a majority of pulling and pushing movements performed in the course of everyday life. The attributes of a well-developed midsection are readily apparent. Plain and simple, your abdominals are the centerpiece of your body; no muscle group gets more attention. And although body fat levels need to be low to see abdominal definition, the often-elusive "six pack" can best be attained by building up the musculature in this region.

Read over the descriptions carefully and scrutinize the photos to ensure proper form. I provide training tips for each of these movements to optimize training performance. Remember that exercises are merely tools for achieving a means to an end—in this case, muscle development. If an exercise does not feel right to you, simply substitute a comparable move.

DUMBBELL PULLOVER

TARGET

This move targets the lats and middle part of the chest.

START

Lie on a flat bench so that your upper back rests on the bench and plant your feet firmly on the floor. Grasp a dumbbell with both hands and raise it directly over your face.

MOVEMENT

Keeping your elbows slightly bent, lower the dumbbell behind your head as far as comfortably possible. When you feel a good stretch in your lats, reverse the direction and return to the start position.

BRAD'S TRAINING TIPS

- Stretch only to the point of comfort—overstretching can lead to shoulder injury.
- Maintain a slight bend in your elbows throughout the move. Do not straighten (extend) your elbows as you lift—this increases triceps activation at the expense of your target muscles.

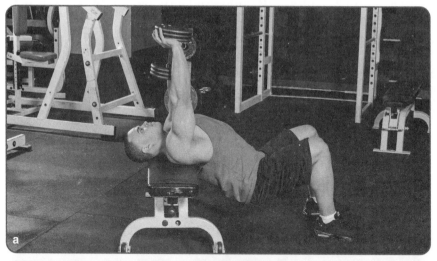

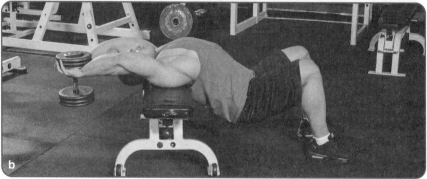

DUMBBELL ONE-ARM ROW

TARGET

This move targets the back muscles and is especially effective for developing the inner-back musculature.

START

Place your left hand and left knee on a flat bench and plant your right foot firmly on the floor. Grasp a dumbbell in your right hand with your palm facing your body and let the dumbbell hang by your side so that your lats achieve a good stretch.

MOVEMENT

Keeping your elbow close to your body, pull the dumbbell up and back until it touches your hip. Contract the muscles in your upper back. Reverse the direction and return to the start position. After you complete the desired number of reps on your right side, reposition yourself on the bench and perform the exercise with your left arm.

BRAD'S TRAINING TIPS

- Keep your back slightly arched and your torso parallel with the floor throughout the move.
- Keep your chin up at all times—this helps prevent rounding of the spine during movement.

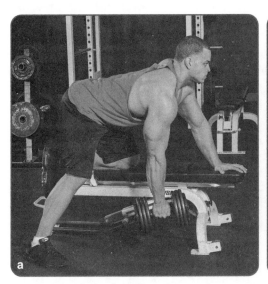
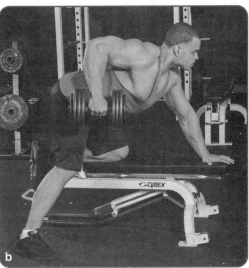

T-BAR ROW

TARGET

This move targets the back muscles.

START

Stand in a T-bar row apparatus with your feet approximately shoulder-width apart. Bend your knees and place the bar between your legs. Grasp the upper portion of the bar with both hands, one hand above the other, and allow the bar to hang down in front of your body so that your lats achieve a good stretch. Bend forward slightly at your hips and hold your core rigid.

MOVEMENT

Keeping your elbows close to your sides, pull the bar up into your midsection as high as comfortably possible. Contract the muscles in your upper back. Reverse the direction and return to the start position.

BRAD'S TRAINING TIPS

- It's extremely important to maintain a slight hyperextension of the lower back. Rounding the spine can result in lumbar injury.
- Keep your head up at all times—this helps prevent rounding of the spine.
- If you wish to perform this exercise at home, wrap a towel around one end of a barbell and wedge the bar in the corner of the room. The towel will help prevent damage to the wall.

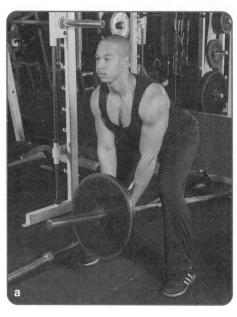 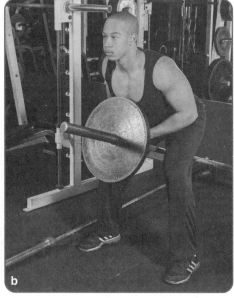

BARBELL REVERSE-GRIP BENT ROW

TARGET

This move targets the back muscles.

START

Grasp a barbell with your hands shoulder-width apart and your palms facing away from your body. Stand with your body angled forward. Bend your knees and slightly arch your lower back. Allow your arms to hang straight down from your shoulders so that your lats achieve a good stretch.

MOVEMENT

Keeping your elbows close to your sides, pull the bar up into your midsection as high as comfortably possible. Contract the muscles in your upper back. Reverse the direction and return to the start position.

BRAD'S TRAINING TIPS

- It's extremely important to maintain a slight hyperextension of the lower back. Rounding the spine can result in lumbar injury.
- Keep your head up at all times—this helps prevent rounding of the spine.

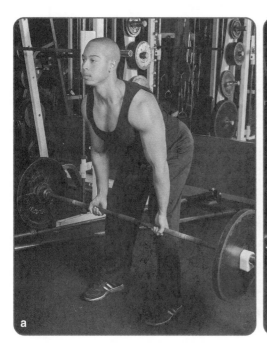
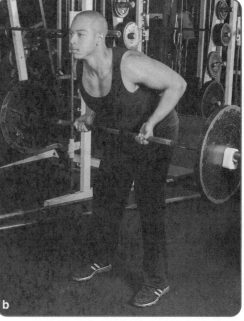

BARBELL OVERHAND BENT ROW

TARGET

This move targets the back muscles.

START

Grasp a barbell with a shoulder-width grip, your palms facing your body. Slightly angle your body forward, bend your knees, and slightly arch your lower back. Allow your arms to hang straight down from your shoulders so that your lats achieve a good stretch.

MOVEMENT

Keeping your elbows close to your sides, pull the bar up into your midsection as high as comfortably possible. Contract the muscles in your upper back. Reverse the direction and return to the start position.

BRAD'S TRAINING TIPS

- It's extremely important to maintain a slight hyperextension of the lower back. Rounding the spine can result in lumbar injury.
- Keep your head up at all times—this helps prevent rounding of the spine.

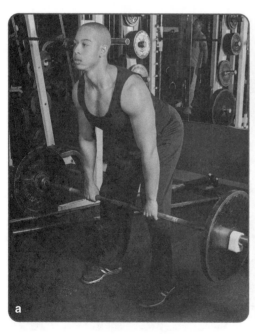
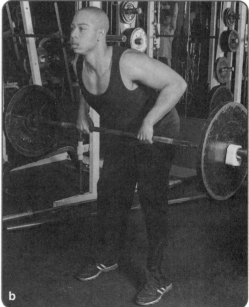

MACHINE CLOSE-GRIP SEATED ROW

TARGET

This move targets the back muscles, particularly the inner musculature of the rhomboids and the middle traps.

START

Sit with your body facing the pad of a seated row machine. Press your chest against the pad and grasp the machine handles, your palms facing each other. Adjust the seat height so that when you grasp the handles, your arms are fully extended and you feel a good stretch in your lats.

MOVEMENT

Keeping your elbows close to your sides and your lower back slightly arched, pull the handles back as far as comfortably possible. Squeeze your shoulder blades together. Reverse the direction and return to the start position.

BRAD'S TRAINING TIP

- Don't swing your body forward at the beginning of the move. This common mistake overstresses the lower-back muscles and interjects unnecessary momentum into the move, which in turn reduces stimulation to the target musculature.

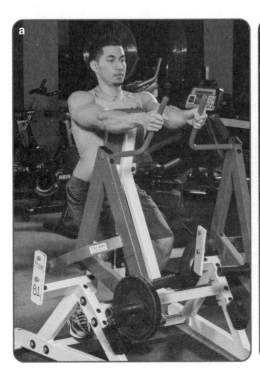
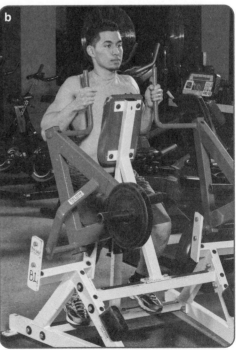

MACHINE WIDE-GRIP SEATED ROW

TARGET

This move targets the back muscles and posterior delts.

START

Sit with your body facing the pad of a seated row machine. Press your chest against the pad and grasp the machine handles with a wide grip. Adjust the seat height so that when you grasp the handles, your arms are fully extended and you feel a good stretch in your lats.

MOVEMENT

Keeping your elbows flared and your lower back slightly arched, pull the handles back as far as comfortably possible. Squeeze your shoulder blades together. Reverse the direction and return to the start position.

BRAD'S TRAINING TIP

- Don't swing your body forward at the beginning of the move. This common mistake overstresses the lower-back muscles and interjects unnecessary momentum into the move, which in turn reduces stimulation to the target musculature.

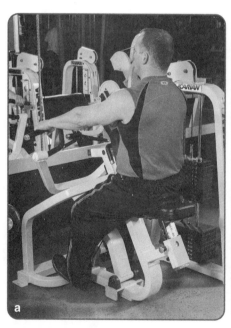 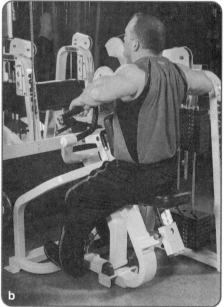

CABLE SEATED ROW

TARGET

This move targets the back muscles, particularly the inner musculature of the rhomboids and the middle traps.

START

With your palms facing each other, grasp the handles of a V-bar attached to a low-pulley apparatus. Sit on the seat (or the floor, depending on the unit) and place your feet against the footplate or a stable part of the unit. Fully straighten your arms so that you feel a good stretch in your lats. Make sure your posture is erect with a slight arch to your lower back.

MOVEMENT

Maintaining a slight bend in your knees, pull the handles in toward your lower abdomen, keeping your elbows close to your sides and your lower back rigid. Squeeze your shoulder blades together when the handles touch your body. Reverse the direction and return to the start position.

BRAD'S TRAINING TIPS

- Don't lean forward on the return—this interjects momentum into the move on the concentric action, reducing tension to the target muscles.
- Never round your spine—this places the discs in a precarious position and can lead to serious injury.
- You can perform this move with a variety of handle attachments, such as the V-bar and the curved bar, based on your personal preference.

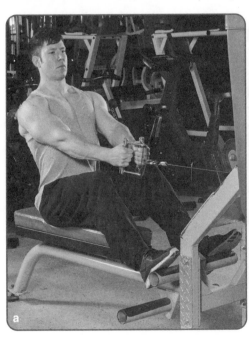
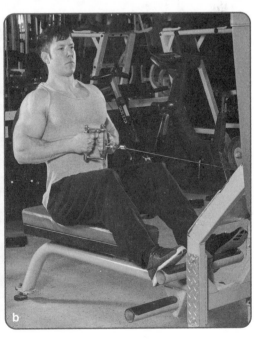

CABLE WIDE-GRIP SEATED ROW

TARGET

This move targets the back muscles and posterior delts.

START

With your palms facing each other, grasp the handles of a wide bar attached to a low-pulley apparatus. Sit on the seat (or the floor, depending on the unit) and place your feet against the footplate or a stable part of the unit. Fully straighten your arms so that you feel a good stretch in your lats. Make sure your posture is erect and slightly arch your lower back.

MOVEMENT

Maintaining a slight bend in your knees, pull the bar in toward your body, keeping your lower back rigid. Squeeze your shoulder blades together when the bar touches your body. Reverse the direction and return to the start position.

BRAD'S TRAINING TIPS

- Don't lean forward on the return—this interjects momentum into the move on the concentric action, reducing tension to the target muscles.
- Never round your spine—this places the discs in a precarious position and can lead to serious injury.

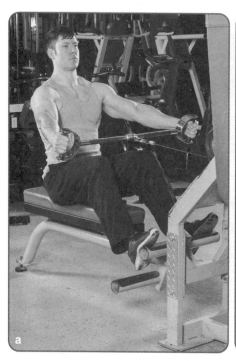
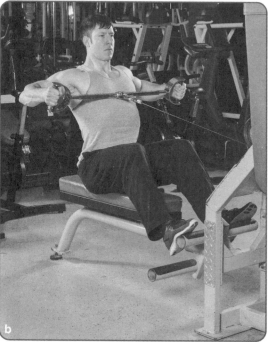

CABLE ONE-ARM STANDING LOW ROW

TARGET

This move targets the back muscles.

START

With your palm facing in, grasp the loop handle of a low pulley with your right hand. Step back from the machine and straighten your right arm so that you feel a good stretch in your right lat. Keep your right leg back and bend your left leg so that your weight is centered slightly forward. Brace your left hand against a sturdy part of the unit for support.

MOVEMENT

Keeping your elbow close to your body, pull the loop handle toward your right side as far as comfortably possible. Contract your right lat. Reverse the direction and return to the start position. After you complete the desired number of reps, repeat the process with your left arm.

BRAD'S TRAINING TIPS

- Don't twist your body to complete the move—this can result in musculoskeletal injury.
- Keep your chin up at all times—this helps prevent rounding of the spine.

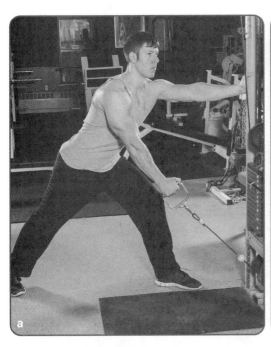
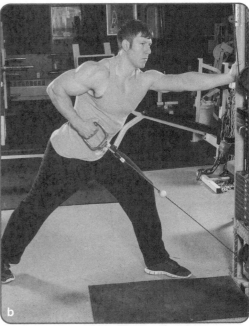

CHIN-UP

TARGET

This move targets the back muscles. Secondary emphasis is on the biceps. A chin-up is generally a bit easier to perform than a pull-up.

START

Grasp a chinning bar with your hands approximately shoulder-width apart and your palms facing your body. Straighten your arms, bend your knees, and cross one foot over the other.

MOVEMENT

Keeping your upper body stable, pull your body up until your chin reaches the bar. Contract your lats. Return your body along the same path to the start position.

BRAD'S TRAINING TIPS

- Don't allow your body to swing—this introduces momentum into the movement, reducing tension to the target muscles.
- The chin-up can be very difficult to execute, especially for those who carry more weight in the lower body. If you can't reach your target rep range, consider using an assisted-chin device (such as a Gravitron) if your gym has one. Alternatively, enlist the help of a partner who can provide assistance by gently pulling up on your ankles as needed.

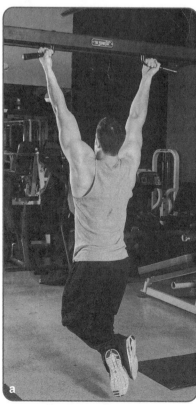
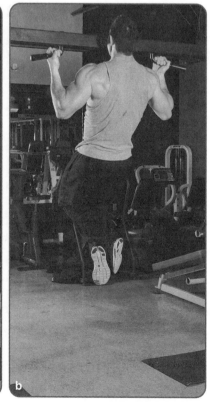

PULL-UP

TARGET

This move targets the back muscles.

START

Grasp a chinning bar with your hands approximately shoulder-width apart and your palms facing away from your body. Straighten your arms, bend your knees, and cross one foot over the other.

MOVEMENT

Keeping your upper body stable, pull your body up until your chin reaches the bar. Contract your lats. Return your body along the same path to the start position.

BRAD'S TRAINING TIPS

- Don't allow your body to swing—this introduces momentum into the movement, reducing tension to the target muscles.

- Avoid taking an overly wide grip because this can shorten range of motion to the point of impairing muscle development. As a general rule, maintain a bilateral width of no more than approximately 1.5 times the length of your clavicle (collarbone).

- The pull-up can be very difficult to execute, especially for those who carry more weight in the lower body. If you can't reach your target rep range, consider using an assisted-chin device (such as a Gravitron) if your gym has one. Alternatively, enlist the help of a partner who can provide assistance by gently pulling up on your ankles as needed.

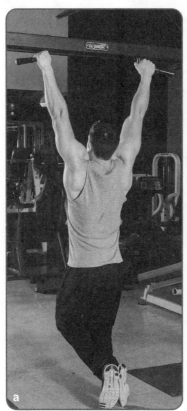
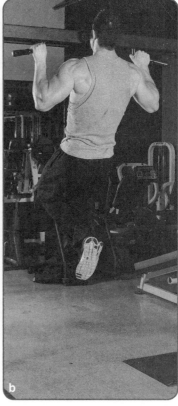

LAT PULL-DOWN

TARGET

This move targets the back muscles, particularly the lats.

START

With your hands approximately shoulder-width apart and your palms facing away from your body, grasp a lat pull-down bar attached to a lat pull-down machine. Secure your knees under the restraint pad and fully straighten your arms so that you feel a good stretch in your lats. Tilt your body back slightly and keep your lower back arched throughout the move.

MOVEMENT

Pull the bar down to your upper chest, angling your elbows slightly back. Squeeze your shoulder blades together. Reverse the direction and return to the start position.

BRAD'S TRAINING TIPS

- Don't lean back more than a few inches—doing so turns the move into a row rather than a pull-down.
- Don't swing your body as you perform the move—this introduces excessive momentum into the lift, reducing tension on the target muscles.

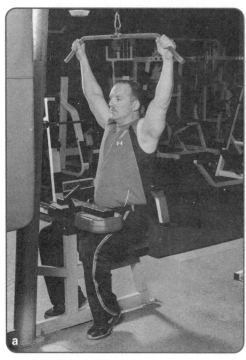 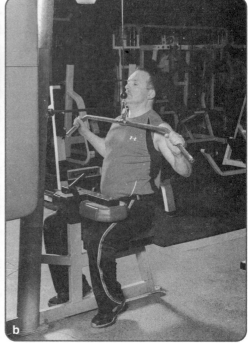

NEUTRAL-GRIP LAT PULL-DOWN

TARGET

This move targets the back muscles.

START

Grasp the handles of a V-bar attached to a lat pull-down machine. Secure your knees under the restraint pad and fully straighten your arms so that you feel a good stretch in your lats. Tilt your body back slightly and keep your lower back arched throughout the move.

MOVEMENT

Pull the handles down to your upper chest, angling your elbows slightly back as you pull. Squeeze your shoulder blades together. Reverse the direction and return to the start position.

BRAD'S TRAINING TIPS

- Don't lean back more than a few inches—doing so turns the move into a row rather than a pull-down.
- Don't swing your body as you perform the move—this introduces excessive momentum into the lift, reducing tension on the target muscles.

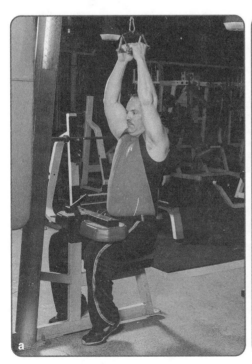
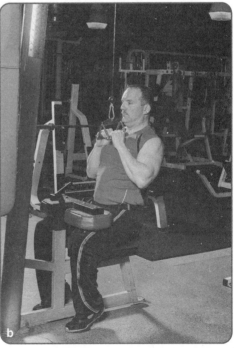

REVERSE-GRIP LAT PULL-DOWN

TARGET

This move targets the back muscles.

START

Grasp a lat pull-down bar with your hands shoulder-width apart and your palms facing your body. Secure your knees under the restraint pad and fully straighten your arms so that you feel a good stretch in your lats. Tilt your body back slightly and keep your lower back arched throughout the move.

MOVEMENT

Pull the bar down to your upper chest, angling your elbows slightly back as you pull. Squeeze your shoulder blades together. Reverse the direction and return to the start position.

BRAD'S TRAINING TIPS

- Don't lean back more than a few inches—doing so turns the move into a row rather than a pull-down.
- Don't swing your body as you perform the move—this introduces excessive momentum into the lift, reducing tension on the target muscles.

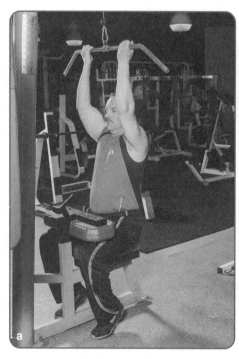 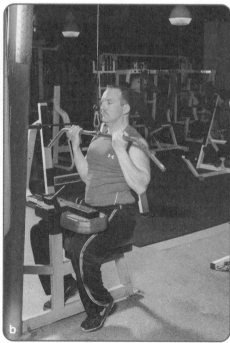

CABLE STRAIGHT-ARM LAT PULL-DOWN

TARGET

This move targets the back muscles, particularly the lats.

START

With your palms facing away from your body, grasp a straight bar attached to a high pulley. Slightly bend your elbows and bring the bar to approximately eye level. Stand with your feet approximately shoulder-width apart. Slightly bend your knees and hold your core rigid.

MOVEMENT

Keeping your upper body erect, pull the bar down until it touches your upper thighs. Contract your back muscles. Reverse the direction and return to the start position.

BRAD'S TRAINING TIP

- You can perform this move with a variety of handle attachments, such as a rope, a curved bar, and loop handles, based on your personal preference.

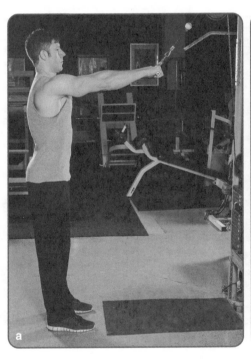
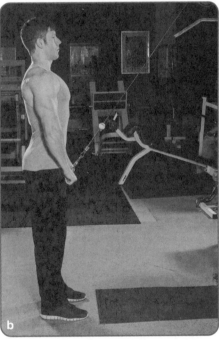

49

CROSS CABLE LAT PULL-DOWN

TARGET

This move targets the back muscles, particularly the lats.

START

Grasp the loop handles of a high-pulley apparatus. Kneel on the floor with your side toward the apparatus and fully extend your arms so that you feel a good stretch in your lat muscles. Face your palms away from your body and slightly arch your lower back.

MOVEMENT

Keeping your body stable, pull the handles down and toward your sides, turning your palms in slightly on the descent. Contract your lats. Reverse the direction and return to the start position.

BRAD'S TRAINING TIP

- Don't allow your elbows to move forward during the move—this changes the plane of movement, altering muscle recruitment.

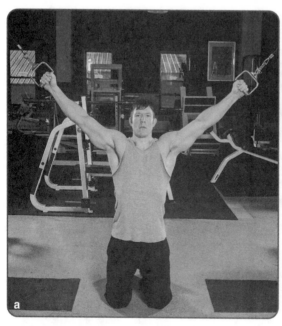
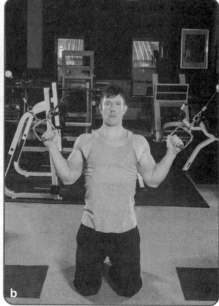

DUMBBELL INCLINE PRESS

TARGET

This move targets the pectorals, particularly the upper part of the chest. It also significantly activates the triceps and front delts.

START

Lie faceup on an incline bench at approximately 30 degrees and plant your feet firmly on the floor. Grasp two dumbbells with your palms facing away from your body. Bring the dumbbells to shoulder level so that they rest just above your armpits.

MOVEMENT

Simultaneously press both dumbbells directly over your chest, moving them in toward each other on the ascent. At the end of the movement, gently touch the sides of the dumbbells together. The weights should be centered over the upper portion of your chest. Contract your chest muscles. Reverse the direction and return to the start position.

BRAD'S TRAINING TIPS

- Keep your elbows flared throughout the move—this helps maintain maximal activation of the pecs.
- As you press the weights, think of moving them in an inverted V pattern to increase range of motion.
- Your body (head, back, and butt) should remain on the bench throughout the performance, without any extraneous movement.
- Don't lock your elbows at the end of the move—this prevents continuous muscle tension.

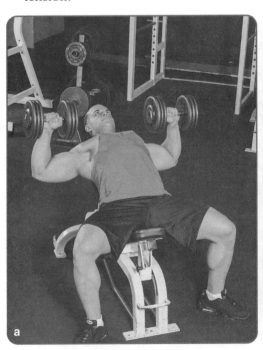 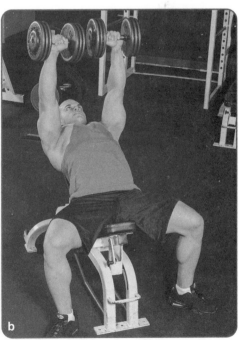

DUMBBELL DECLINE PRESS

TARGET

This move targets the pectorals, particularly the lower fibers of the muscle. It also significantly activates the front delts and triceps.

START

Lie faceup on a decline bench and secure your feet in the restraint pad. Grasp two dumbbells with your palms facing away from your body. Bring the dumbbells to shoulder level so that they rest just above your armpits.

MOVEMENT

Simultaneously press both dumbbells directly over your chest, moving them in toward each other on the ascent. At the end of the movement, gently touch the sides of the dumbbells together. The weights should be centered over the lower portion of your chest. Contract your chest muscles. Reverse the direction and return to the start position.

BRAD'S TRAINING TIPS

- Keep your elbows flared throughout the move—this helps maintain maximal activation of the pecs.
- As you press the weights, think of moving them in an inverted V pattern to increase range of motion.
- Your body (head, back, and butt) should remain on the bench throughout the performance, without any extraneous movement.
- Don't lock your elbows at the end of the move—this prevents continuous muscle tension.

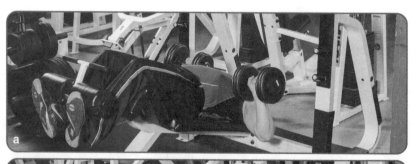

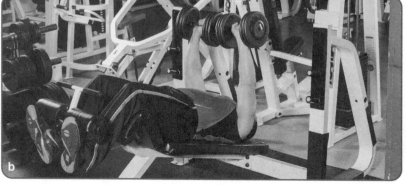

DUMBBELL CHEST PRESS

TARGET

This move targets the pectorals, particularly the sternal part of the chest. Secondary emphasis is on the front delts and triceps.

START

Lie faceup on a flat bench and plant your feet firmly on the floor. Grasp two dumbbells with your palms facing away from your body. Bring the dumbbells to shoulder level so that they rest just above your armpits.

MOVEMENT

Simultaneously press both dumbbells directly over your chest, moving them in toward each other on the ascent. At the end of the movement, gently touch the sides of the dumbbells together. The weights should be centered over the middle portion of your chest. Contract your chest muscles. Reverse the direction and return to the start position.

BRAD'S TRAINING TIPS

- Keep your elbows flared throughout the move—this helps maintain maximal activation of the pecs.
- As you press the weights, think of moving them in an inverted V pattern to increase range of motion.
- Your body (head, back, and butt) should remain on the bench throughout the performance, without any extraneous movement.
- Don't lock your elbows at the end of the move—this prevents continuous muscle tension.

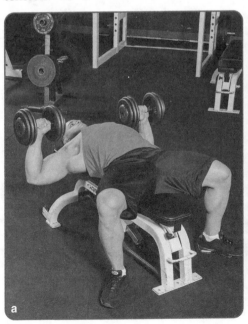
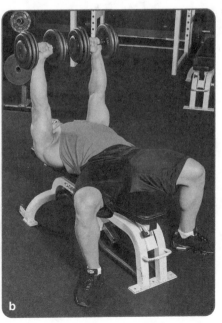

BARBELL INCLINE PRESS

TARGET

This move targets the pectorals, particularly the upper part of the chest. It also significantly activates the triceps and front delts.

START

Lie faceup on an incline bench set at approximately 30-40 degrees and plant your feet firmly on the floor. Grasp a barbell with your hands about shoulder-width apart and bring it down to the upper aspect of your chest.

MOVEMENT

Press the bar directly over your upper chest, moving it in a straight line into the air. At the end of the movement, the bar should be centered over the upper portion of your chest. Contract your chest muscles. Return the bar along the same path to the start position.

BRAD'S TRAINING TIPS

- Keep your elbows flared throughout the move.
- Your body (head, back, and butt) should remain on the bench throughout the performance, without any extraneous movement.
- Don't lock your elbows at the end of the move—this prevents continuous muscle tension.

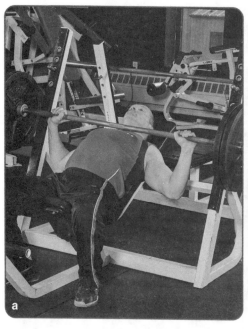
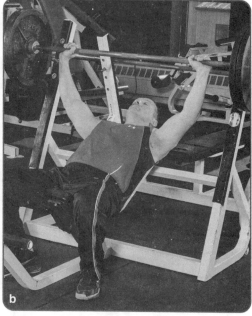

BARBELL CHEST PRESS

TARGET

This move targets the pectorals, particularly the sternal part of the chest. It also significantly works the triceps and front delts.

START

Lie faceup on a flat bench and plant your feet firmly on the floor. Grasp a barbell with your hands approximately shoulder-width apart and bring it down to the middle of your chest.

MOVEMENT

Press the bar directly over your chest, moving it in a straight line into the air. At the end of the movement, the bar should be centered over the middle portion of your chest. Contract your chest muscles. Return the bar along the same path to the start position.

BRAD'S TRAINING TIPS

- Keep your elbows flared throughout the move.
- Your body (head, back, and butt) should remain on the bench throughout the performance, without any extraneous movement.
- Don't lock your elbows at the end of the move—this prevents continuous muscle tension.

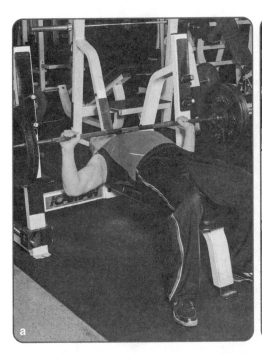 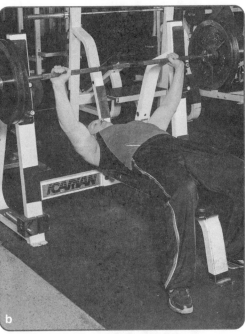

BARBELL DECLINE PRESS

TARGET

This move targets the pectorals, particularly the lower part of the chest. It also significantly works the triceps and front delts.

START

Lie faceup on a decline bench and secure your feet under the restraint pad. Grasp a barbell with your hands approximately shoulder-width apart and bring it down to the middle of your chest.

MOVEMENT

Press the bar directly over your chest, moving it in a straight line into the air. At the end of the movement, the bar should be centered over the lower portion of your chest. Contract your chest muscles. Return the bar along the same path to the start position.

BRAD'S TRAINING TIPS

- Keep your elbows flared throughout the move.
- Your body (head, back, and butt) should remain on the bench throughout the performance, without any extraneous movement.
- Don't lock your elbows at the end of the move—this prevents continuous muscle tension.

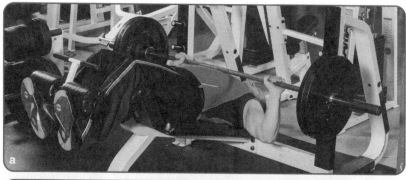

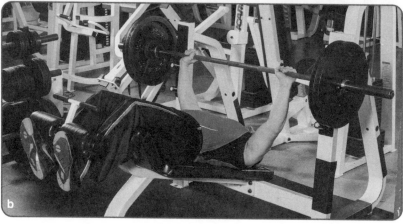

MACHINE INCLINE PRESS

TARGET

This move targets the pectorals, particularly the upper portion. Secondary emphasis is on the front delts and triceps.

START

Lie back on the seat of an incline press machine set at approximately 40 degrees (if the bench is adjustable) and align your upper chest with the handles on the machine. Grasp the handles with your hands shoulder-width apart and your palms facing away from your body. Flare your elbows.

MOVEMENT

Keeping your back against the support pad, press the handles forward, stopping just before you fully lock your elbows. Contract your chest muscles. Reverse the direction and return to the start position.

BRAD'S TRAINING TIPS

- Depending on the machine, you may be able to adjust the incline of the bench to varying degrees to optimally target the upper chest in the incline press. Make sure that the action moves in line with the upper portion of your chest. A muscle always contracts maximally when the action is carried out in line with its fibers.

- Keep your elbows flared as you lift—allowing them to move forward changes the scope of the exercise.

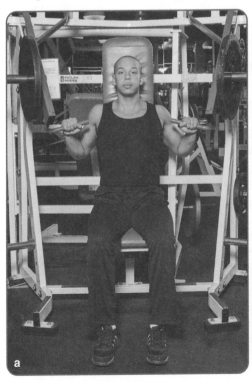
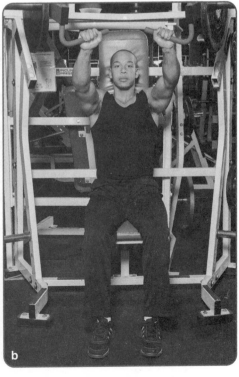

MACHINE CHEST PRESS

TARGET

This move targets the chest muscles, particularly the sternal portion. Secondary emphasis is on the front delts and triceps.

START

Sit in a chest press machine and align your upper chest with the handles on the machine. Grasp the handles with your hands about shoulder-width apart and your palms facing away from your body.

MOVEMENT

Press the handles forward, stopping just before you fully lock your elbows. Contract your chest muscles. Reverse the direction and return to the start position.

BRAD'S TRAINING TIP

- Keep your elbows flared as you lift so that they remain approximately parallel with the floor. Allowing them to move downward changes the plane of the exercise and alters muscle recruitment.

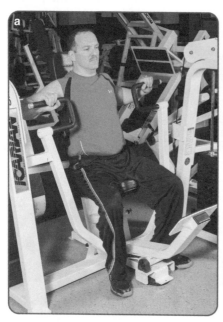 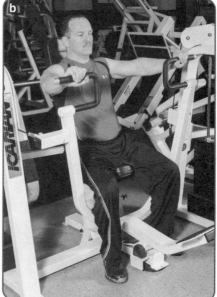

DUMBBELL FLAT FLY

TARGET

This move targets the pectorals, primarily the sternal fibers. It provides better isolation for the chest muscles than the flat press. Secondary emphasis is on the front delts.

START

Lie faceup on a flat bench and plant your feet firmly on the floor. Grasp two dumbbells and bring them out to your sides with a slight bend in your elbows. Face your palms in and toward the ceiling, and hold your upper arms roughly parallel with the level of the bench.

MOVEMENT

Raise the weights up in a semicircular motion and gently touch the weights together at the top of the move. At the end of the move, the dumbbells should be centered over the upper portion of your chest. Contract your chest muscles. Return the weights along the same path to the start position.

BRAD'S TRAINING TIPS

- Keep your arms rounded throughout the move—do not straighten your elbows.
- As you lift the weights, it can be helpful to think of hugging a beach ball to maintain the semicircular motion.
- Your body (head, back, and butt) should remain on the bench throughout the performance, without any extraneous movement.
- Avoid overstretching in the start position—this can cause injury.

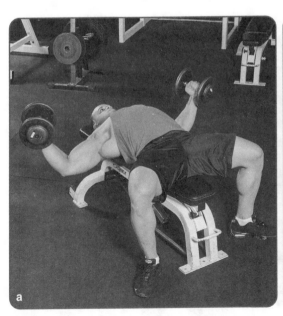
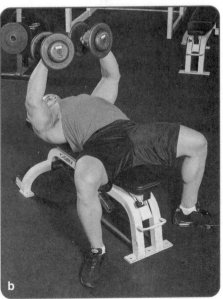

DUMBBELL INCLINE FLY

TARGET

This move targets the pectorals, particularly the upper fibers. It provides better isolation for the chest muscles than the incline press. Secondary emphasis is on the front delts.

START

Lie faceup on an incline bench set at approximately 40 degrees and plant your feet firmly on the floor. Grasp two dumbbells and bring them out to your sides with a slight bend in your elbows. Face your palms in and toward the ceiling, and hold your upper arms roughly parallel with the level of the bench.

MOVEMENT

Raise the weights upward in a semicircular motion and gently touch the weights together at the top of the move. At the end of the move, the dumbbells should be centered over the upper portion of your chest. Contract your chest muscles. Return the weights along the same path to the start position.

BRAD'S TRAINING TIPS

- Keep your arms rounded throughout the move—do not straighten your elbows.
- As you lift the weights, it can be helpful to think of hugging a beach ball to maintain the semicircular motion.
- Your body (head, back, and butt) should remain on the bench throughout the performance, without any extraneous movement.
- Avoid overstretching in the start position—this can cause injury.

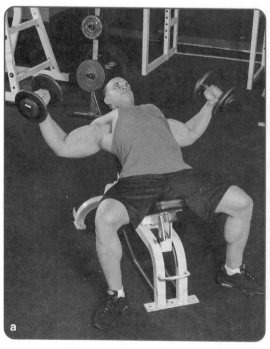
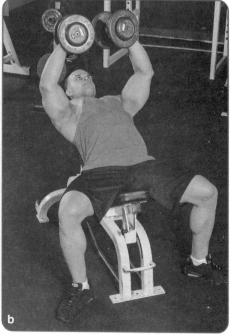

PEC DECK FLY

TARGET

This move targets the chest muscles. Secondary emphasis is on the front delts.

START

Grasp the handles of a pec deck machine with your palms facing away from your body. Slightly bend your elbows and keep your back rigid throughout the move.

MOVEMENT

Bring the handles together simultaneously and gently touch your hands together directly in front of your chest. Contract your pectoral muscles. Reverse the direction and return to the start position.

BRAD'S TRAINING TIP

- Several types of pec deck units exist. They all accomplish the same task, so use whatever version is available to you or whichever unit suits your preference.

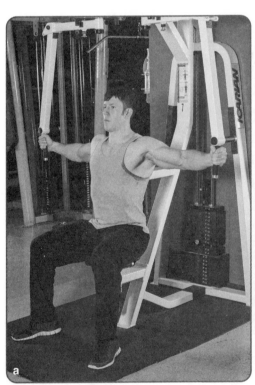
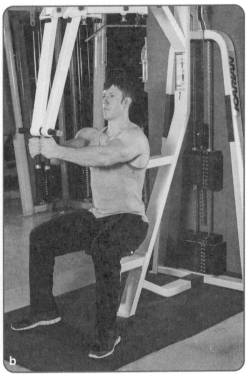

CABLE FLY

TARGET

This move targets the chest muscles, particularly the sternal portion. Secondary emphasis is on the front delts.

START

Grasp the handles of a high-pulley apparatus. Stand with your feet about shoulder-width apart in a staggered stance and slightly bend your torso forward at the waist. Slightly bend your arms and hold them out to the sides so that they are approximately parallel with the floor.

MOVEMENT

Keeping your upper torso and your core rigid, pull both handles down and across your body, creating a semicircular movement. Bring your hands together at the level of your waist and squeeze your chest muscles so that you feel a contraction in the midline area. Reverse the direction and allow your hands to return along the same path to the start position.

BRAD'S TRAINING TIPS

- Your elbows should remain slightly bent and fixed throughout the move—don't flex or extend them at any time. That alteration turns the exercise into a pressing movement rather than a fly.
- As you lift, it can be helpful to think of hugging a beach ball to maintain the semicircular motion.

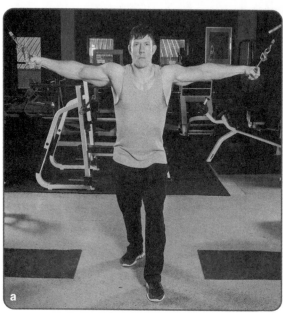 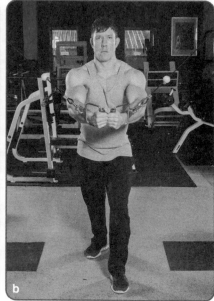

CHEST DIP

TARGET

This move targets the pectorals, particularly the lower fibers. Secondary emphasis is on the front delts and triceps.

START

Place your hands on the parallel bars of a dip apparatus with your palms facing your sides. Hold your arms straight and slightly bend your knees and hips.

MOVEMENT

Leaning your torso forward, bend your arms and allow your elbows to flare out to the sides. Lower your body as far as comfortably possible. Feel a stretch in your pectoral muscles. Reverse the direction by straightening your arms until you reach the start position.

BRAD'S TRAINING TIPS

- If you cannot attain the necessary number of reps, enlist a partner to hold your feet and provide assistance. Alternatively, you can use an assisted-dip device (such as a Gravitron) to facilitate performance.
- To increase the level of difficulty, place a dumbbell between your ankles.

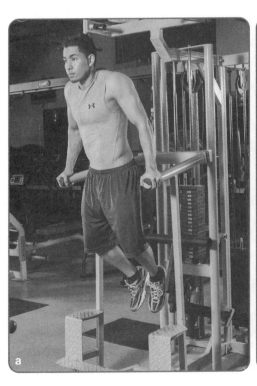
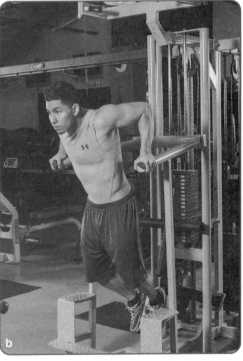

CRUNCH

TARGET

This move targets the abs, particularly the upper abdominal region.

START

Lie faceup on the floor. Bend your knees and plant your feet. Press your lower back into the floor and fold your hands across your chest.

MOVEMENT

Keeping the lower portion of your back flat on the floor with the lumbar spine held neutral, raise your shoulders up and forward toward your chest. Contract your abdominal muscles. Reverse the direction and return to the start position.

BRAD'S TRAINING TIPS

- Don't allow your upper back to touch the floor when lowering—doing so reduces tension to the abs.
- If the move becomes easy, hold a weighted object such as a dumbbell or medicine ball against your chest.
- Never place your hands behind your head—this encourages pulling on the neck muscles, which can potentially lead to injury.

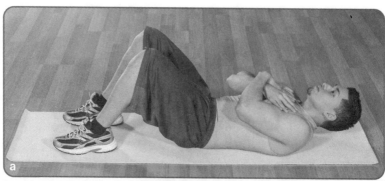

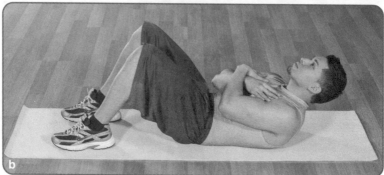

REVERSE CRUNCH

TARGET

This move targets the abs, particularly the lower abdominal region.

START

Lie faceup on the floor with your hands at your sides. Curl your knees into your abdomen and lift your butt so that it is slightly off the floor.

MOVEMENT

Keeping your upper back pressed into the floor, raise your butt as high as comfortably possible so that your pelvis tilts toward your chest. Contract your abs. Reverse the direction and return to the start position.

BRAD'S TRAINING TIPS

- Keep your upper torso completely stable—the only parts of your body that should move are your hips and lumbar spine.
- Don't just push your butt up in the air. Rather, focus on pulling your pelvis toward your belly button. This forces the lower portion of the abs to do more of the work. It's a short range of motion that, when done properly, really hits the target muscle.
- Don't allow your butt to touch the floor when lowering—doing so reduces tension to the abs.
- If the move becomes easy, place a medicine ball between your thighs.

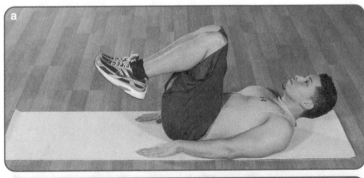

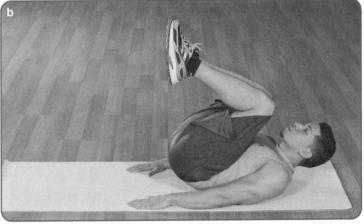

BICYCLE CRUNCH

TARGET

This move targets the abs.

START

Sit on the floor with your torso and legs angled at about 30 degrees. Curl your hands and place them at your ears.

MOVEMENT

Bring your left knee up toward your right elbow and try to touch them to one another. As you return your left leg and right elbow to the start position, bring your right leg toward your left elbow in the same manner. Continue this movement, alternating between right and left sides, as if pedaling a bike.

BRAD'S TRAINING TIPS

- Never place your hands behind your head—this encourages pulling on the neck muscles, which can potentially lead to injury.
- Avoid the temptation to speed up on this move. As with all exercise, perform in a smooth, controlled manner with a strong mind–muscle connection for optimal results.

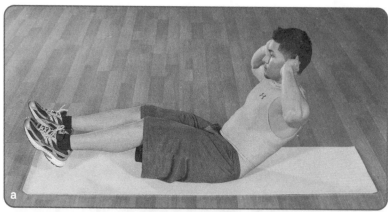

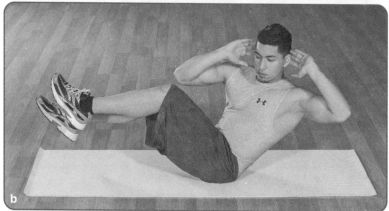

ROMAN CHAIR SIDE CRUNCH

TARGET

This move targets the obliques.

START

Lie on your right side on the top of a Roman chair with your feet secure under the restraint pad. Place your left fingertips by your left temple and keep your elbows wider than your body. Keep your bottom elbow flared, your hand on your hip.

MOVEMENT

Raise your top elbow so that your trunk laterally flexes as far as comfortably possible. Contract your obliques. Return along the same path to the start position. After you complete the desired number of reps, repeat the process on the opposite side.

BRAD'S TRAINING TIP

- If you have trouble maintaining stability, hold on to the hip pad with your bottom hand.

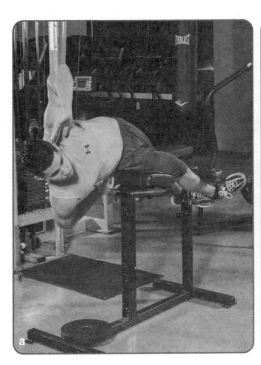 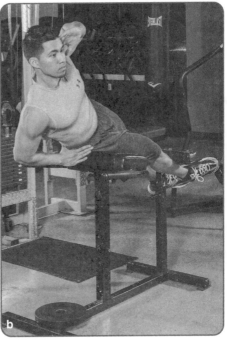

STABILITY BALL ABDOMINAL CRUNCH

TARGET

This move targets the abs.

START

Sit on top of a stability ball and place your feet shoulder-width apart. Walk your feet forward until the ball firmly supports your lower back. Place your hands on your chest and lower your upper back and shoulders onto the ball.

MOVEMENT

Lift your upper back and shoulders off the ball as far as comfortably possible. Contract your abs. Return along the same path to the start position.

BRAD'S TRAINING TIPS

- Sitting higher on the ball (i.e., your butt on top of the ball) makes the exercise more difficult; sitting lower on the ball makes it easier.
- Keep your lower back on the ball at all times. Lifting your lower back engages the hip flexors, reducing stress on the target muscles.
- Keep your hips anchored so that you move over the ball and the ball does not roll under you.
- If the move becomes easy, hold a weighted object such as a dumbbell or medicine ball against your chest.

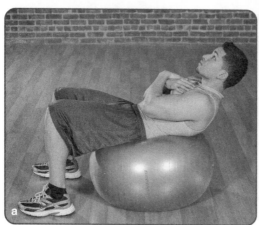 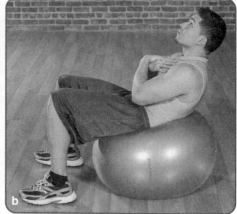

CABLE ROPE KNEELING CRUNCH

TARGET

This move targets the abs, particularly the upper portion.

START

Face a high-pulley apparatus and kneel down to a kneeling position. Grasp the ends of a rope (or the loop handles) attached to the pulley. Place your elbows near your ears and hold your torso upright.

MOVEMENT

Keeping your lower back rigid, curl your shoulders down, bringing your elbows down toward your knees. Contract your abs. Uncurl your body and return to the start position.

BRAD'S TRAINING TIP

- Curl only from your upper torso—your hips and lower back should remain fixed throughout the move. This maintains tension on the abs and removes activation of the hip flexors.

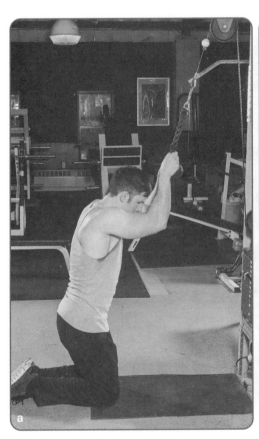
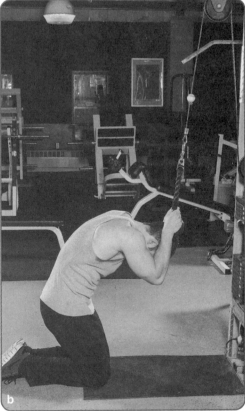

CABLE ROPE KNEELING TWISTING CRUNCH

TARGET

This move targets the abs and obliques.

START

Face a high-pulley apparatus and kneel down to a kneeling position. Grasp the ends of a rope (or the loop handles) attached to the pulley. Place your elbows near your ears and hold your torso upright.

MOVEMENT

Keeping your lower back rigid, curl your shoulders down, twisting your body to the right as you bring your elbows toward your right knee. Contract your abs. Uncurl your body and return to the start position. Alternate twisting to the right and to the left for the desired number of reps.

BRAD'S TRAINING TIP

- Curl only from your upper torso—your hips and lower back should remain fixed throughout the move. This maintains tension on the target muscles and removes activation of the hip flexors.

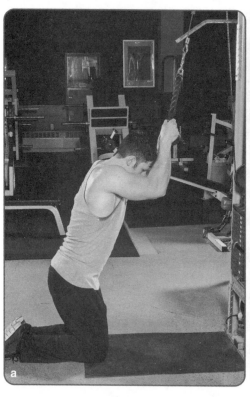
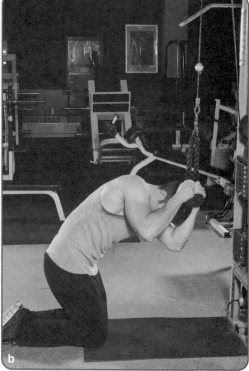

TOE TOUCH

TARGET

This move targets the abs, particularly the upper abdominal region.

START

Lie faceup on the floor. Hold your arms and legs straight in the air, perpendicular to your body.

MOVEMENT

Keeping the lower portion of your back flat on the floor with the lumbar spine held neutral, curl your torso up and forward, moving your hands as close to your toes as comfortably possible. Contract your abs. Reverse the direction and return to the start position.

BRAD'S TRAINING TIPS

* Keep your head in line with your torso at all times—unwanted movement can potentially injure the cervical region.
* For added intensity, hold a weighted object such as a dumbbell or medicine ball in your hands.

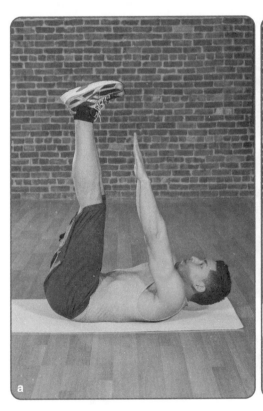
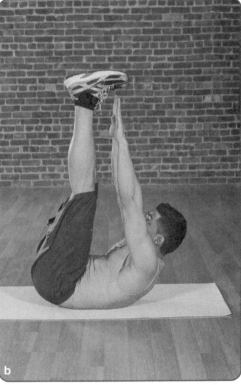

PLANK

TARGET

This move targets the entire core.

START

Lie facedown with your palms or forearms on the floor and your spine in a neutral position. Place your feet together.

MOVEMENT

Keeping your body as straight as possible, lift your body up, balancing your weight on your forearms and toes. Maintain this position for as long as possible. Return to the start position. As your core strength increases, progressively challenge yourself to maintain the plank position for longer periods of time.

BRAD'S TRAINING TIPS

- Use your core strength to keep your body rigid—don't allow any part of your body to sag at any time.
- Aim to work up to a hold of more than 60 seconds.
- To increase the level of difficulty, perform the move with one leg off the floor.
- For added intensity, perform the move on an unstable device such as a BOSU or a small stability ball.

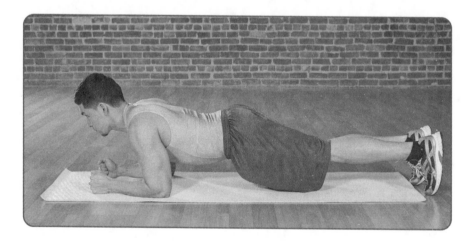

SIDE BRIDGE

TARGET

This move targets the entire core, particularly the obliques.

START

Lie on your right side with your right forearm on the floor. Hold your legs straight and stack one foot on top of the other.

MOVEMENT

Straighten your right arm, keeping it in line with your shoulder, and place your left hand on your left hip so that your elbow is bent approximately 90 degrees. Hold this position for as long as possible. Repeat the process on the opposite side.

BRAD'S TRAINING TIPS

- Use your core strength to keep your body rigid—don't allow any part of your body to sag at any time.
- Balance on the side of your foot, not the sole.
- Aim to work up to a hold of more than 60 seconds.
- To increase the level of difficulty, perform the move with your braced arm straight and your palm flat on the floor.
- For added intensity, perform the move on an unstable device such as a BOSU or a small stability ball.

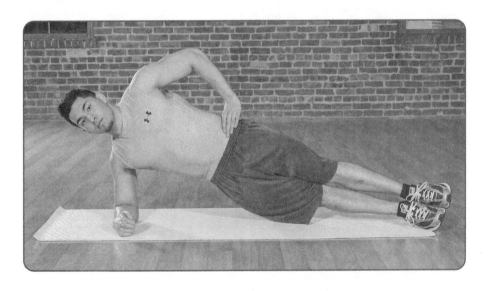

HANGING KNEE RAISE

TARGET

This move targets the abs.

START

Grasp a chinning bar with your hands approximately shoulder-width apart and your palms facing away from your body. Bend your knees and stabilize your torso.

MOVEMENT

Keeping your knees bent, raise your thighs upward, lifting your butt so that your pelvis tilts toward your abdomen. Contract your abs. Reverse the direction and return your legs to the start position. For increased intensity, straighten your legs while performing the move.

BRAD'S TRAINING TIPS

- Focus on pulling your pelvis up and back so that it approaches your belly button. This forces the lower portion of the abs to do more of the work.
- If you have trouble holding your body weight, consider using hanging ab straps.
- Keep your upper torso motionless throughout the move—don't swing to complete a repetition.

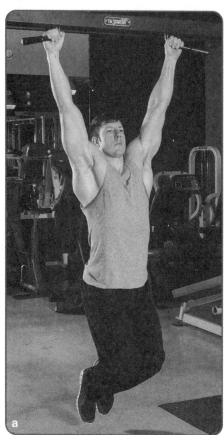 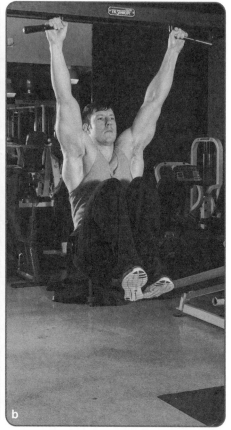

RUSSIAN TWIST

TARGET

This move targets the obliques.

START

Sit on the floor and rigidly hold your torso about 45 degrees to the floor. Grasp a medicine ball and hold it close to your torso. Bend your knees about 40 degrees and lift your feet slightly off the floor.

MOVEMENT

Keeping your lower body stable, twist your torso to one side as far as comfortably possible. Rotate back to center and repeat the process to the other side.

BRAD'S TRAINING TIPS

- Move only at the core—not at your shoulders or hips.
- Keep your eyes on your hands at all times to enhance core rotation.

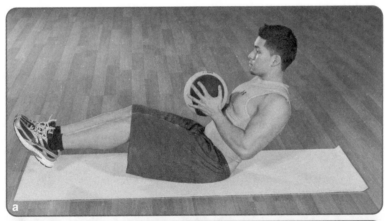

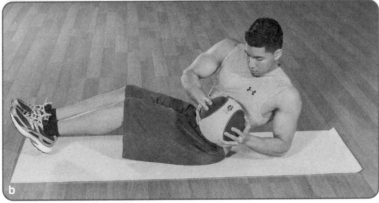

CABLE SIDE BEND

TARGET

This move targets the obliques.

START

With your left hand, grasp a loop handle attached to a low-pulley apparatus. Stand with your left side facing the machine and take a small step away from the unit so that there is tension in the cable. Keep your feet shoulder-width apart. Hold your torso erect and slightly bend your knees.

MOVEMENT

Keeping your core rigid, bend your torso as far to the right as comfortably possible. Contract your obliques. Return along the same path to the start position. After you complete the desired number of reps, repeat the process on the opposite side.

BRAD'S TRAINING TIPS

- The movement should take place solely at your waist—your hips shouldn't move at all during the movement.
- Your upper body should remain in the same plane at all times—don't sway forward or backward.

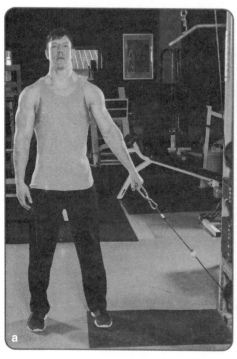 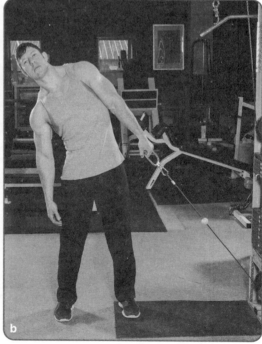

CABLE WOOD CHOP

TARGET

This move targets the obliques.

START

Grasp the ends of a cable attached to a cable-pulley apparatus. If possible, adjust the cable so that it is at chest height. (If the machine is not adjustable, you can perform the move from the high- or low-pulley positions.) Stand with your right side facing the machine and with your feet shoulder-width apart. Hold your torso erect and slightly bend your knees. Extend your arms across your body to the right as far as comfortably possible.

MOVEMENT

Keeping your lower body stable, pull the cable up and across your torso to the left (as if you were chopping wood). Contract your obliques. Return along the same path to the start position. After you complete the desired number of reps, repeat the process on the opposite side.

BRAD'S TRAINING TIP

- To keep constant tension on the obliques, make sure the action takes place at your waist—not your hips.

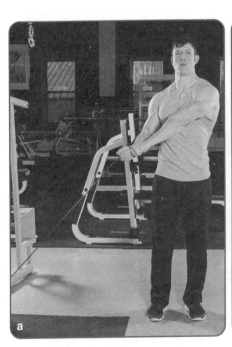
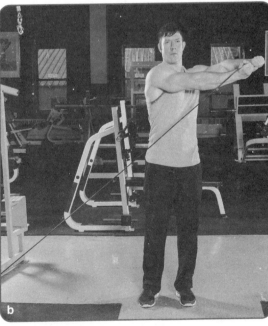

BARBELL ROLLOUT

TARGET

This move targets the abs.

START

Load a pair of small plates (weights that are 5 pounds [2.3 kg] work well) onto the ends of a barbell. Grasp the middle of the bar with your hands approximately shoulder-width apart and your palms facing away from your body. Kneel down so that your shoulders are just behind the bar. Keep your upper back straight and hold your butt up.

MOVEMENT

Keeping your knees fixed on the floor and your arms rigid, roll the bar forward as far as comfortably possible without allowing your body to touch the floor. Reverse the direction by forcefully contracting your abs and return along the same path to the start position.

BRAD'S TRAINING TIPS

- To maximize activation of the abdominal musculature, the action should take place solely at the waist—not the hips.
- The contraction happens as you pull back to the start position—the rollout stretches the abs.
- You can use various wheel-based devices for the rollout if it suits your preference.

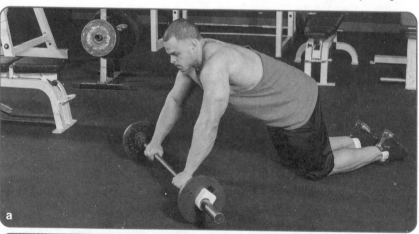

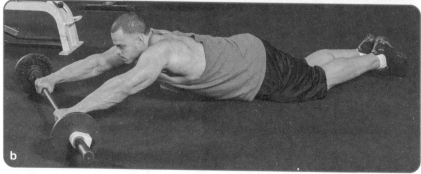

EXERCISES FOR THE SHOULDERS AND ARMS

This chapter describes and illustrates exercises for the muscles of the shoulders and arms. Because these muscle groups reside on the extremities, they are generally more visible than the musculature of the torso and lower body. Hence, people tend to place increased emphasis on their development. Well-developed shoulders are essential for achieving the classic V taper. The biceps and triceps are the "show muscles" of the body that epitomize strength.

Read over the descriptions carefully and scrutinize the photos to ensure proper form. I provide training tips for each of these movements to optimize training performance. Remember that exercises are merely tools for achieving a means to an end—in this case, muscle development. If an exercise does not feel right to you, simply substitute a comparable move.

MILITARY PRESS

TARGET

This move targets the shoulders, particularly the front delts. Secondary emphasis is on the upper trapezius and triceps.

START

Assume a shoulder-width stance in front of a power rack. Grasp a barbell and bring it to the level of your upper chest with your palms facing away from your body.

MOVEMENT

Press the barbell directly up and over your head. Contract your delts at the top of the move. Reverse the direction and return the bar along the same path to the start position.

BRAD'S TRAINING TIPS

- Keep your elbows forward, not flared, throughout the move to maintain movement in the sagittal plane.
- If you don't have access to a power rack, you will need to clean the bar to shoulder level.
- You can perform the exercise seated, which helps to reduce the use of the lower musculature during performance and thus increases stimulation of the target musculature.

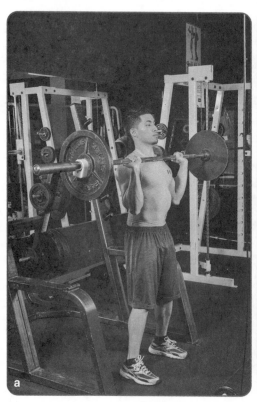
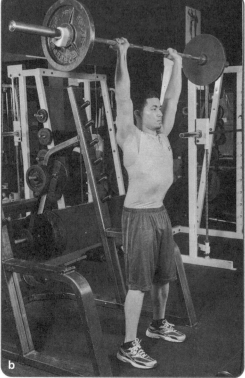

DUMBBELL SHOULDER PRESS

TARGET

This move targets the deltoids, particularly the front delts. Secondary emphasis is on the upper trapezius and triceps.

START

Sit on the edge of a flat bench or chair. Grasp two dumbbells and bring the weights to shoulder level with your palms facing away from your body.

MOVEMENT

Press the dumbbells directly up and in. Touch the weights together directly over your head. Contract your delts. Return the dumbbells along the same arc to the start position.

BRAD'S TRAINING TIPS

- Don't arc the weights outward as you press—this reduces exercise efficiency and increases stress on the connective tissue in the shoulder joint. Instead, think of pressing the weights in an inverted V pattern.
- You can perform this exercise standing if desired, but avoid engaging your lower body in the movement to maintain maximal tension on the target musculature.

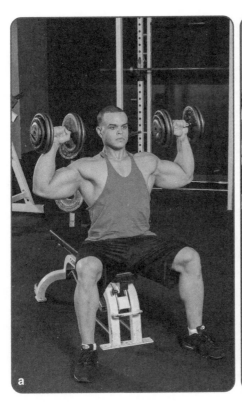
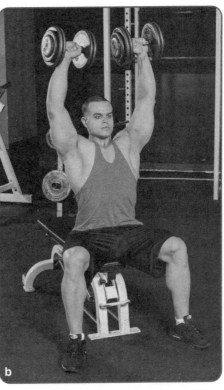

MACHINE SHOULDER PRESS

TARGET

This move targets the deltoids, particularly the front delts. Secondary emphasis is on the upper trapezius and triceps.

START

Sit upright in the seat of a shoulder press machine and support your back on the pad. Grasp the handles of the machine with your palms facing away from your body and your elbows flared out to the sides. Adjust the seat height so that the handles are approximately in line with your shoulders.

MOVEMENT

Keeping your elbows flared, press the handles directly up and over your head. Contract your delts at the top of the move. Return the handles to the start position.

BRAD'S TRAINING TIPS

- Don't lock your elbows at the top of the move—doing so reduces tension to the target muscles.
- Keep your elbows flared to the sides as you lift—allowing them to move forward changes the plane of the exercise.

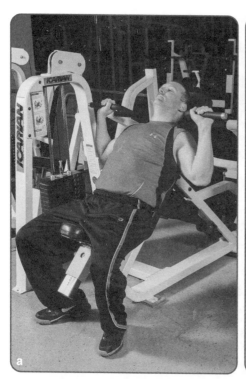 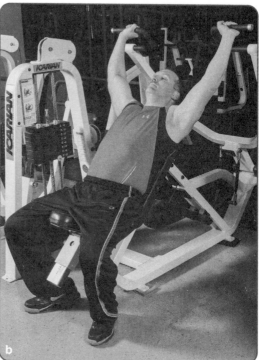

DUMBBELL LATERAL RAISE

TARGET

This move targets the middle delts.

START

Sit on the end of a flat bench with your back straight. Grasp two dumbbells and allow them to hang by your hips.

MOVEMENT

Keeping your elbows slightly bent, raise the dumbbells up and out to your sides until they reach shoulder level. At the top of the movement, the rears of the dumbbells should be slightly higher than the fronts. Contract your delts. Return the weights along the same path to the start position.

BRAD'S TRAINING TIPS

- Think of pouring a cup of milk as you lift—this keeps maximum tension on the middle delts.
- Raise the weight only up to shoulder level—going higher than this can cause shoulder impingement.
- You can also perform this move from a standing position if desired, but avoid engaging your lower body in the movement to maintain maximal tension on the target musculature.

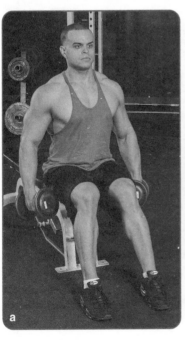
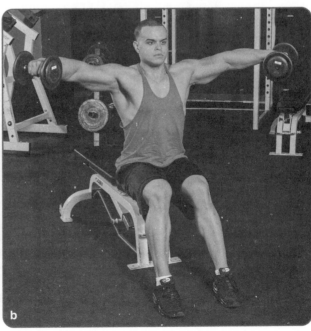

MACHINE LATERAL RAISE

TARGET

This move targets the middle delts.

START

Sit in a lateral raise machine and press your torso against the chest pad. Adjust the seat so that your forearms align with the restraint pad. Place your forearms under the restraint pad and firmly grasp the attached handles with your palms facing each other.

MOVEMENT

Keeping your elbows flared, raise your upper arms up and out to the sides until they reach shoulder level. Contract your delts. Return along the same path to the start position.

BRAD'S TRAINING TIP

- Raise the weight only up to shoulder level—going higher than this can cause shoulder impingement.

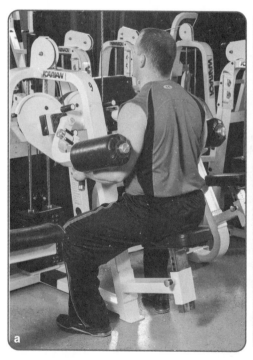
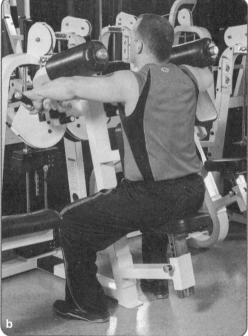

CABLE LATERAL RAISE

TARGET

This move targets the middle delts.

START

With your right hand, grasp a loop handle attached to a low-pulley apparatus. Stand with your left side facing the machine, your feet approximately shoulder-width apart, and your torso erect. Slightly bend your knees and hold your core rigid.

MOVEMENT

Maintain a slight bend in your elbow throughout the movement. Raise the handle across your body, up, and out to the side until it reaches the level of your shoulder. Contract your delts at the top of the movement. Return the handle to the start position. After you complete the desired number of reps, repeat the process on the opposite side.

BRAD'S TRAINING TIPS

- Think of pouring a cup of milk as you lift. Your pinky should be slightly higher than your thumb at the top of the move—this keeps maximum tension on the middle delts.

- Raise the weight only up to shoulder level—going higher than this can cause shoulder impingement.

- Keep your upper arms directly out to the sides at all times—allowing them to gravitate inward switches the emphasis to the front delts at the expense of the middle delts.

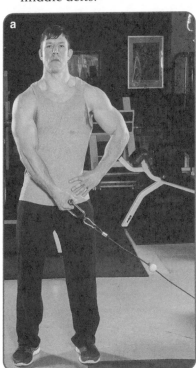 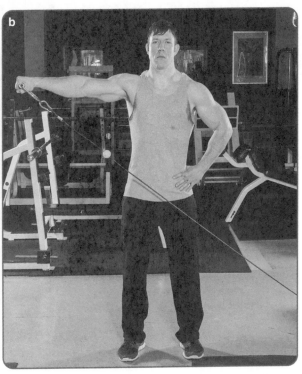

DUMBBELL BENT REVERSE FLY

TARGET

This move targets the posterior (rear) delts. I prefer this move to the standing version because it places less stress on the lower back.

START

Grasp two dumbbells and sit on the edge of a bench or chair. Bend your torso forward so that it is almost parallel with the floor. Allow the dumbbells to hang down behind the legs.

MOVEMENT

Keeping your elbows slightly bent, raise the dumbbells up and out to your sides until they are parallel with the floor. Contract your delts at the top of the movement. Return the dumbbells to the start position.

BRAD'S TRAINING TIPS

- Don't swing your body to complete a repetition—this takes work away from the target muscles.
- Avoid the natural tendency to bring your elbows in toward the body as you lift. Hold your elbows out and away from the body throughout the move to keep maximal tension on the rear delts.

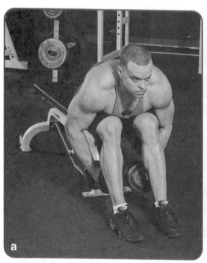 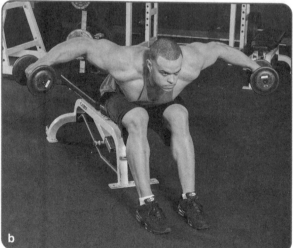

MACHINE REAR DELT FLY

TARGET

This move targets the posterior (rear) delts.

START

Sit facing forward in a pec deck machine and press your chest up against the pad. Slightly bend your elbows and grasp the machine handles with your palms facing down.

MOVEMENT

Keeping your arms parallel with the floor, pull the handles back in a semicircular arc until they are approximately perpendicular to your torso. Contract your rear delts. Reverse the direction and return the handles to the start position.

BRAD'S TRAINING TIP

- Keep your arms parallel with the floor throughout the move. If you are not able to keep your arms parallel, adjust the seat height accordingly.

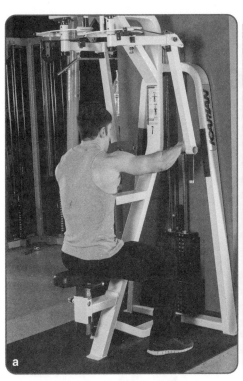
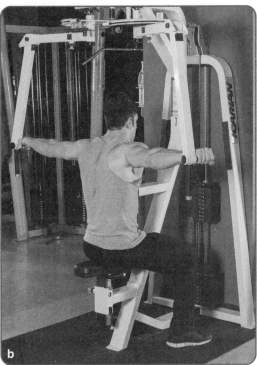

CABLE REVERSE FLY

TARGET

This move targets the posterior (rear) delts.

START

Assume a shoulder-width stance in front of a cable-pulley apparatus. Grasp the end of the left cable with your right hand and grasp the end of the right cable with your left hand. Keeping your torso rigid, take a couple steps back so that there is tension in the pulleys.

MOVEMENT

Keeping your arms slightly bent, simultaneously pull the cables out and back in a circular movement as far as comfortably possible. Contract your posterior delts. Return to the start position.

BRAD'S TRAINING TIPS

- Don't straighten your arms as you perform the move—this causes the triceps to assist in the movement at the expense of the target musculature.
- Don't swing your body to complete a repetition—this takes work away from the target muscles.

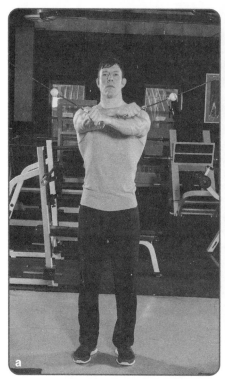
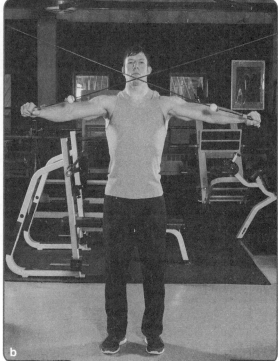

CABLE KNEELING REVERSE FLY

TARGET

This move targets the posterior (rear) delts.

START

With your right hand, grasp a loop handle attached to a low-pulley apparatus. Kneel on your hands and knees. Stabilize your torso with your left arm. Position your right arm under your chest and slightly bend your right elbow.

MOVEMENT

Keep your working arm slightly bent and your core rigid throughout the movement. Raise the handle out to your right side until your arm is parallel with the floor. Contract your delts at the top of the movement. Return the handle to the start position. After you complete the desired number of reps, repeat the process on your left side.

BRAD'S TRAINING TIP

- Avoid the natural tendency to bring your elbows in toward your body as you lift. Hold your elbows away from your body throughout the movement to keep maximal tension on the rear delts.

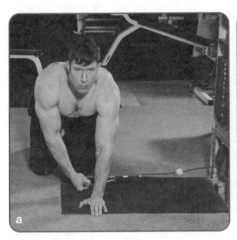
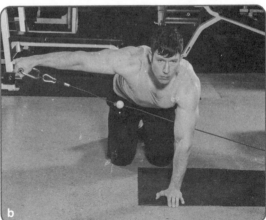

BARBELL UPRIGHT ROW

TARGET

This move targets the middle delts. Secondary emphasis is on the biceps.

START

Grasp a barbell with a shoulder-width grip. Allow your arms to hang down from your shoulders with your palms facing your body. Assume a comfortable stance and bend your knees slightly.

MOVEMENT

Raise the bar up along the line of your body until your upper arms approach shoulder level, keeping your elbows higher than your wrists at all times. Contract your delts. Reverse the direction and lower the bar along the same path to the start position.

BRAD'S TRAINING TIPS

- Don't lift your elbows beyond a position that is parallel with the floor. Doing so can lead to shoulder impingement, which injures the rotator cuff.
- Keep the bar as close to your body as possible throughout the movement.

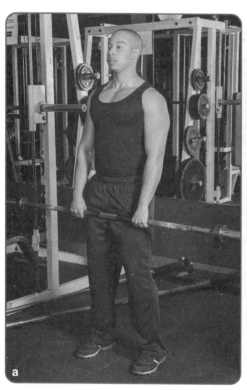 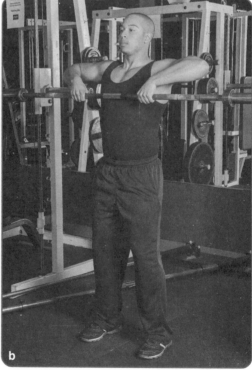

CABLE UPRIGHT ROW

TARGET

This move targets the middle delts. Secondary emphasis is on the biceps and upper trapezius.

START

Grasp the ends of a rope (or the loop handles) attached to a low-pulley apparatus. Stand with your feet shoulder-width apart and your torso erect. Slightly bend your knees and hold your core rigid. Allow your arms to hang down from your shoulders in front of your body without locking your elbows.

MOVEMENT

Pull the rope up along the line of your body until your upper arms approach shoulder level. Keep your elbows higher than your wrists at all times. Contract your delts. Reverse the direction and lower the rope along the same path to the start position.

BRAD'S TRAINING TIPS

- Initiate the action by lifting the elbows, not the wrists, to ensure optimal stimulation of the target muscles.
- Don't lift your elbows beyond a position that is parallel with the floor. Doing so can lead to shoulder impingement, which injures the rotator cuff.
- Keep your hands as close to your body as possible throughout the entire move.
- Perform the move with a straight bar or EZ-curl bar if you desire.

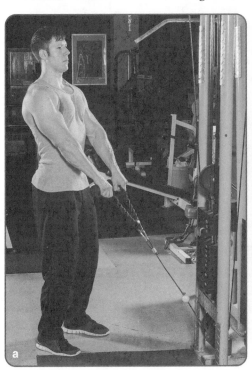
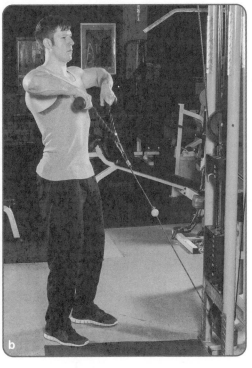

DUMBBELL STANDING BICEPS CURL

TARGET

This move targets the biceps.

START

Assume a shoulder-width stance and slightly bend your knees. Grasp a pair of dumbbells and allow them to hang at your sides with your palms facing forward.

MOVEMENT

Press your elbows into your sides and keep them immobile throughout the move. Curl the dumbbells up toward your shoulders. Contract your biceps at the top of the move. Reverse the direction and return to the start position.

BRAD'S TRAINING TIPS

- If desired, begin with your palms facing your sides and actively supinate your hands as you lift.
- Keep your wrists straight as you lift—don't roll them to complete the move.
- You can also perform this move from a seated position, which can help to reduce contributions from extraneous muscles.

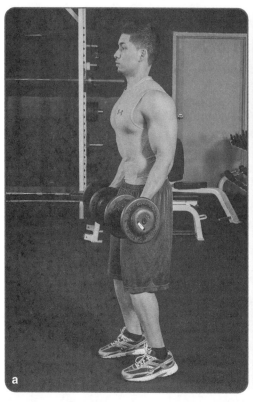 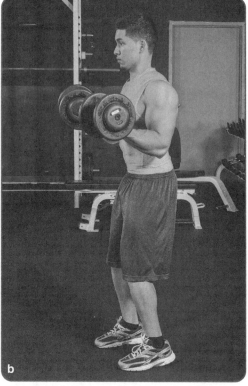

DUMBBELL INCLINE BICEPS CURL

TARGET

This move targets the biceps. Because the shoulders are kept in an extended position, this move is especially effective for targeting the long head.

START

Lie faceup on an incline bench set at 40 degrees. Grasp two dumbbells and allow the weights to hang behind your body with your palms facing forward.

MOVEMENT

Keeping your upper arms immobile, curl the dumbbells up toward your shoulders. Contract your biceps. Reverse the direction and return the weights to the start position.

BRAD'S TRAINING TIPS

- Keep your elbows back throughout the movement so that the shoulders are maintained in an extended position—this keeps maximal tension on the biceps, especially the long head.

- Keep your wrists straight as you lift—don't roll them to complete the move.

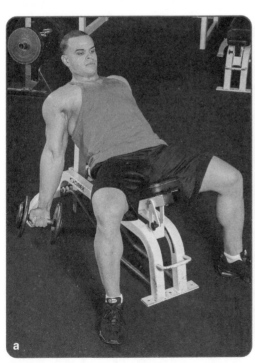
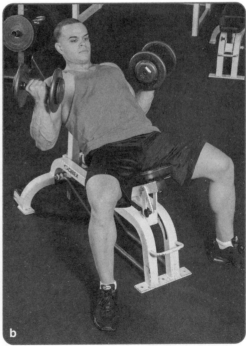

DUMBBELL PREACHER CURL

TARGET

This move targets the biceps, particularly the short head.

START

Grasp a dumbbell with your left hand. Place the upper portion of your left arm on a preacher curl bench and extend your left forearm just short of locking out the elbow.

MOVEMENT

Keeping your upper arm pressed to the bench, curl the dumbbell up toward your shoulder. Contract your biceps. Reverse the direction and return the weight to the start position. After you complete the desired number of reps, repeat the process on your right side.

BRAD'S TRAINING TIPS

- Fully brace your upper arm on the bench—there should be no space between your arm and the bench.
- Keep your wrists straight as you lift—don't roll them to complete the move.
- If you do not have access to a preacher curl bench, use an incline bench instead.

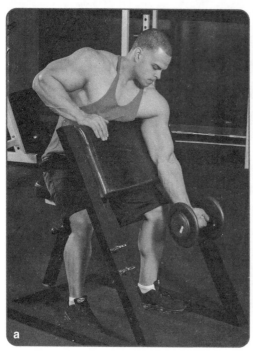
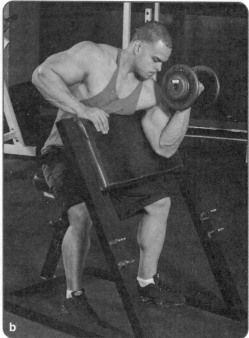

BARBELL PREACHER CURL

TARGET

This move targets the biceps, particularly the short head.

START

Grasp a barbell with both hands. Place the upper portions of your arms on a preacher curl bench and extend your forearms just short of locking out the elbow.

MOVEMENT

Keeping your upper arms pressed to the bench, curl the bar up toward your shoulders. Contract your biceps. Reverse the direction and return the bar to the start position.

BRAD'S TRAINING TIPS

- Fully brace your upper arms on the bench—there should be no space between your arms and the bench.
- Keep your wrists straight as you lift—don't roll them to complete the move.
- You can perform this move with either a straight bar or an EZ-curl bar. The EZ-curl bar can help alleviate pressure on your wrists.

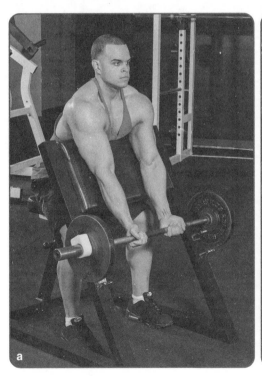

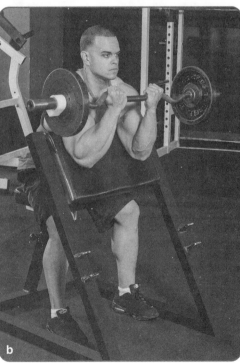

MACHINE PREACHER CURL

TARGET

This move targets the biceps, particularly the short head.

START

Sit upright in a curl machine. Adjust the seat so that your armpits align with the top of the pad. Grasp the machine handles with your palms facing your body and place the backs of your arms on the pad.

MOVEMENT

Keeping your torso erect, raise the handles toward your shoulders as far as comfortably possible. Contract your biceps. Reverse the direction and return to the start position.

BRAD'S TRAINING TIP

- To maintain optimal tension on the biceps, press your upper arms on the pads throughout the entire movement.

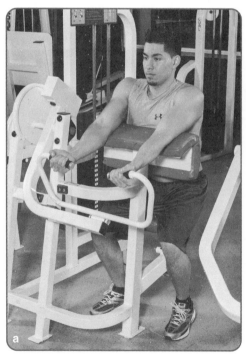
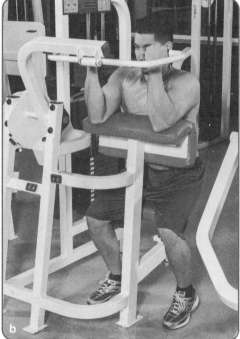

CONCENTRATION CURL

TARGET

This move targets the biceps, particularly the short head.

START

Sit on the edge of a flat bench with your legs wide apart. Grasp a dumbbell in your right hand and brace your right triceps on the inside of your right thigh. Straighten your arm so that it hangs down near the floor.

MOVEMENT

Curl the weight up and in along the line of your body. Contract your biceps at the top of the move. Reverse the direction and return to the start position. After you complete the desired number of reps, repeat the process on your left side.

BRAD'S TRAINING TIPS

- Brace your exercising arm on your inner thigh at all times. If you struggle to complete a rep, use your opposite hand to assist the move—don't swing your exercising arm.

- Keep your wrists straight as you lift—don't roll them to complete the move.

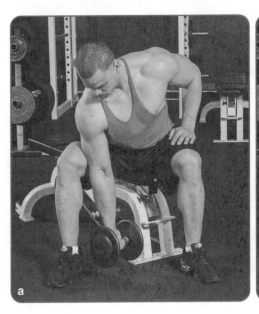
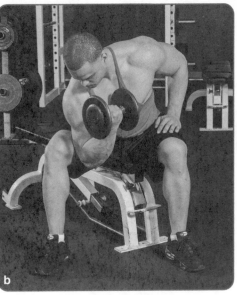

DUMBBELL STANDING HAMMER CURL

TARGET

This move targets the upper arms, particularly the brachialis and brachioradialis.

START

Assume a shoulder-width stance and slightly bend your knees. Grasp a pair of dumbbells and allow them to hang at your sides with your palms facing each other.

MOVEMENT

Keeping your elbows pressed into your sides, curl the dumbbells up toward your shoulders. Contract your biceps at the top of the move. Reverse the direction and return to the start position.

BRAD'S TRAINING TIP

• Keep your wrists straight as you lift—don't roll them to complete the move.

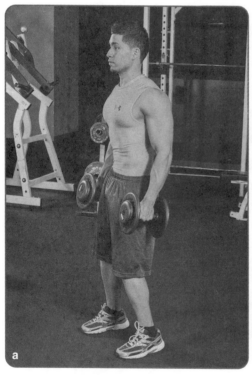
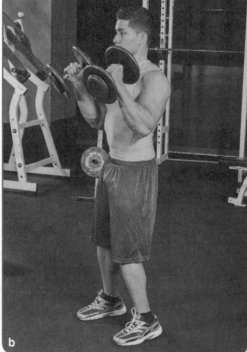

BARBELL CURL

TARGET

This move targets the biceps.

START

Assume a comfortable stance and bend your knees slightly. Grasp a barbell with a shoulder-width grip, your palms facing up.

MOVEMENT

Keeping your upper arms pressed into your sides, curl the bar up toward your shoulders. Contract your biceps at the top of the move. Reverse the direction and return to the start position.

BRAD'S TRAINING TIPS

- Keep your upper arms motionless throughout the move—all activity takes place at the elbow.
- You can perform this move with either a straight bar or an EZ-curl bar. The EZ-curl bar can help alleviate pressure on your wrists.

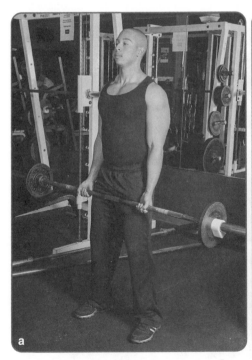
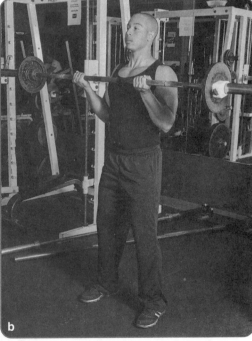

BARBELL DRAG CURL

TARGET

This move targets the biceps, particularly the long head.

START

Grasp a barbell with a shoulder-width grip, your palms facing up. Allow the bar to hang in front of your body and slightly bend your elbows. Assume a comfortable stance and slightly bend your knees.

MOVEMENT

Keeping your upper arms close to your sides and immobile throughout the move, bring your elbows behind your body, curling the bar along the line of your torso up toward your shoulders. Contract your biceps. Reverse the direction and return to the start position.

BRAD'S TRAINING TIPS

• Move your elbows back as you lift—this keeps maximum tension on the long head.

• You can perform this move with either a straight bar or an EZ-curl bar. The EZ-curl bar can help alleviate pressure on your wrists.

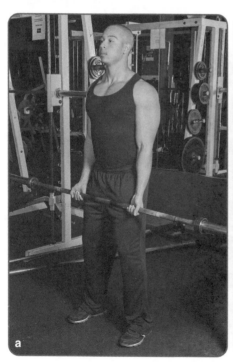

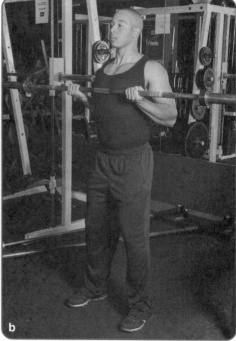

CABLE ROPE HAMMER CURL

TARGET

This move targets the upper arms, particularly the brachialis and brachioradialis.

START

Grasp both ends of a rope (or loop handles) attached to a low-pulley apparatus. Press your elbows into your sides with your palms facing each other. Stand with your feet shoulder-width apart and your torso erect. Slightly bend your knees and hold your core rigid.

MOVEMENT

Keeping your upper arms immobile throughout the move, curl the rope up toward your shoulders. Contract your biceps at the top of the move. Reverse the direction and return to the start position.

BRAD'S TRAINING TIPS

- Don't allow your upper arms to move forward as you lift—this brings your shoulders into the movement at the expense of your arm muscles.

- Keep your wrists straight as you lift—don't roll them to complete the move.

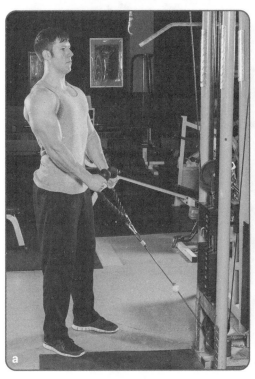
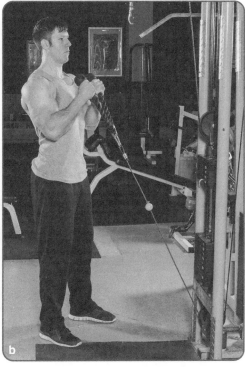

CABLE CURL

TARGET

This move targets the biceps.

START

Grasp a straight bar attached to a low-pulley apparatus. Press your elbows into your sides with your palms facing up. Stand with your feet shoulder-width apart and your torso erect. Slightly bend your knees and hold your core rigid.

MOVEMENT

Keeping your upper arms immobile throughout the move, curl the bar up toward your shoulders. Contract your biceps. Reverse the direction and return to the start position.

BRAD'S TRAINING TIPS

- Keep your wrists straight as you lift—don't roll them.
- Don't allow your upper arms to move forward as you lift—this brings your shoulder into the movement at the expense of your arm muscles.

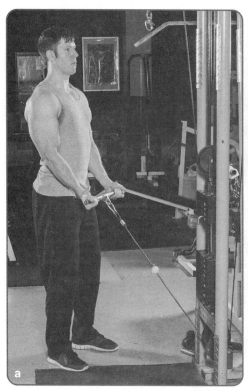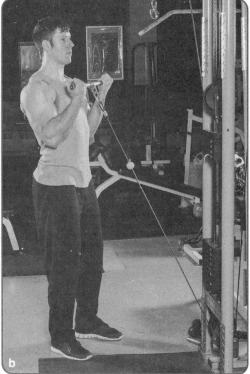

CABLE ONE-ARM CURL

TARGET

This move targets the biceps.

START

With your right hand, grasp a loop handle attached to a low-pulley apparatus. Press your right elbow into your right side with your palm down. Stand with your feet shoulder-width apart and your torso erect. Slightly bend your knees and hold your core rigid.

MOVEMENT

Keeping your upper arm immobile throughout the move and your palm turning to face up, curl the handle up toward your shoulder. Contract your biceps. Reverse the direction and return to the start position. After you complete the required number of reps, repeat the process on your left side.

BRAD'S TRAINING TIPS

- Keep your wrists straight as you lift—don't roll them.
- Don't allow your upper arm to move forward as you lift—this brings your shoulder into the movement at the expense of your arm muscles.

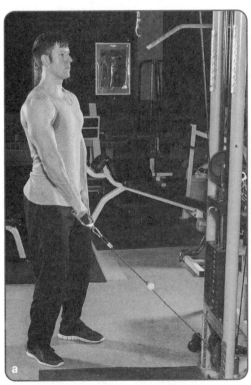
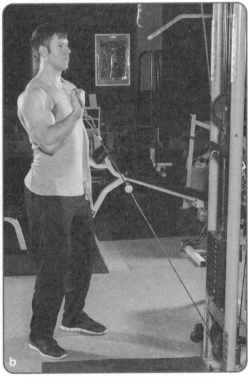

DUMBBELL OVERHEAD TRICEPS EXTENSION

TARGET

This move targets the triceps, particularly the long head.

START

Grasp the stem of a dumbbell with both hands. Sit on the edge of a flat bench or chair and bring the dumbbell overhead. Bend your elbows and allow the weight to hang down behind your head as far as comfortably possible.

MOVEMENT

Keeping your elbows back and pointed toward the ceiling, straighten your arms. Contract your triceps. Reverse the direction and lower the weight along the same path to the start position.

BRAD'S TRAINING TIPS

- Keep your elbows pinned to your ears as you lift—if your elbows flare, you'll reduce the stress on the triceps.
- If you have difficulty maintaining an erect posture, place the bench in an upright position and brace your back against the pad.
- If desired, perform this exercise one arm at a time. This allows you to focus on each arm individually and may alleviate stress on the elbow joint.

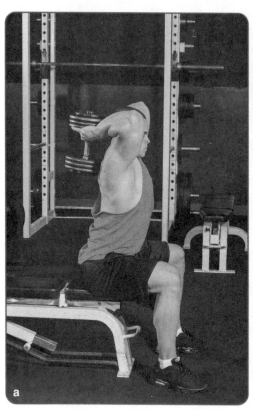 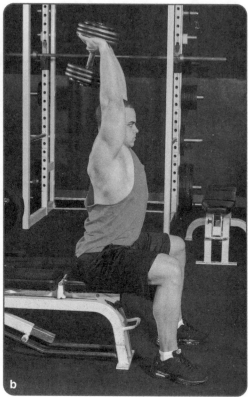

CABLE ROPE OVERHEAD TRICEPS EXTENSION

TARGET

This move targets the triceps, particularly the long head.

START

Grasp the ends of a rope (or loop handles) attached to a high-pulley apparatus and face away from the machine. Press your elbows close to your ears and bend your elbows. Allow your hands to hang behind your head with your palms facing each other as far as comfortably possible. Bring one foot in front of the other. Stand with your torso erect and bend your knees slightly.

MOVEMENT

Keeping your elbows close to your ears, straighten your arms as fully as possible. Contract your triceps. Reverse the direction and return the weight along the same path to the start position.

BRAD'S TRAINING TIPS

- Pin your elbows to your ears as you lift—if your elbows flare, you'll reduce the stress on the triceps.
- Keep your upper arms completely stationary throughout the move—any forward movement diminishes tension on the triceps.
- If desired, perform this exercise one arm at a time. This allows you to focus on each arm individually and may alleviate stress on the elbow joint.

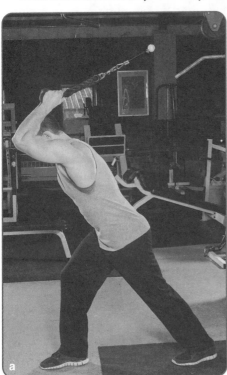 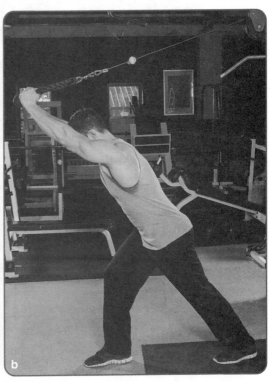

105

SKULL CRUSHER

TARGET

This move targets the triceps.

START

Lie faceup on a flat bench and plant your feet firmly on the floor. Grasp a barbell with your palms facing up and straighten your arms so that the barbell is directly centered over your chest. Your arms should be perpendicular to your body.

MOVEMENT

Keeping your elbows in and pointed toward the ceiling, lower the barbell until it reaches a point just above the level of your forehead. Reverse the direction and press the barbell up until it reaches the start position.

BRAD'S TRAINING TIPS

- Pin your elbows to your ears as you lift—if your elbows flare, you'll reduce the stress on the triceps.
- You can perform this exercise one arm at a time with a dumbbell. This allows you to focus on each arm individually and may alleviate stress on the elbow joint.

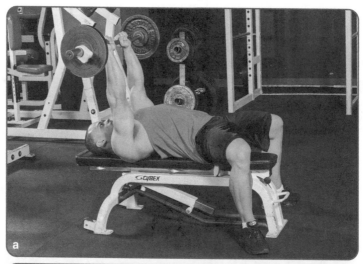

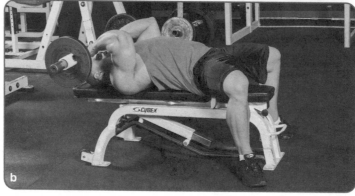

MACHINE SKULL CRUSHER

TARGET

This move targets the triceps.

START

Sit in the machine and align the seat so that your upper arms rest comfortably on the pad and are approximately parallel with the ground. Grasp the handles of the machine with your palms facing one another.

MOVEMENT

Keeping your torso erect and your elbows in, push the handles down until your arms fully straighten. Contract your triceps. Reverse the direction and return to the start position.

BRAD'S TRAINING TIP

- Keep your upper arms in contact with the pad at all times throughout the move. Otherwise, secondary muscles will take over the exercise.

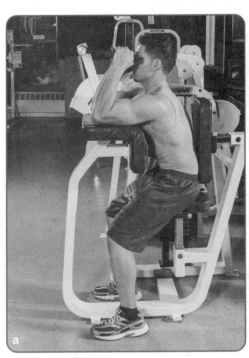 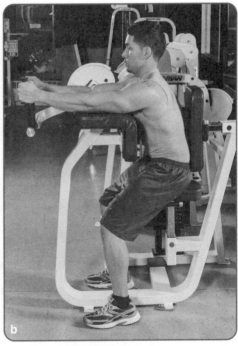

DUMBBELL TRICEPS KICKBACK

TARGET

This move targets the triceps, particularly the middle and lateral heads.

START

Stand with your body bent forward so that it is almost parallel with the floor. Grasp a dumbbell with your left hand and press your left arm against your side. Bend your left elbow so that it forms a 90-degree angle. If desired, you can brace your alternate arm on a bench for stability.

MOVEMENT

With your palm facing your body, straighten your arm until it is parallel with the floor. Reverse the direction and return the weight to the start position. After you complete the desired number of reps, repeat the process on your right side.

BRAD'S TRAINING TIPS

- Don't let your upper arm sag down as you lift—this reduces the effects of gravity and thus diminishes tension to the target muscles.

- Don't flick your wrist at the top of the movement—this common error fatigues the forearm muscles before sufficiently fatiguing the triceps and reduces the effectiveness of the move.

- Arch your back slightly throughout the movement. Never round your spine—this increases stress on the lumbar area and could lead to injury.

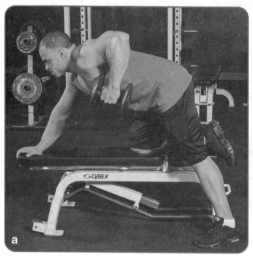
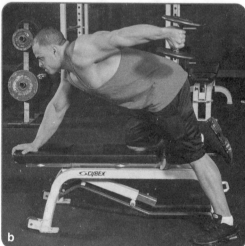

CABLE TRICEPS KICKBACK

TARGET

This move targets the triceps, particularly the middle and lateral heads.

START

Grasp a loop handle attached to a low-pulley apparatus. Bend your torso forward so that it is roughly a 40-degree angle with the floor. Press your right arm against your side with your palm facing back. Bend your right elbow 90 degrees. Stand with your feet approximately shoulder-width apart in a staggered stance and your back straight. Bend your knees slightly and hold on to a sturdy part of the machine with your left hand for support.

MOVEMENT

Keeping your upper arm immobile, straighten your arm until it is parallel with the floor. Reverse the direction and return to the start position. After you complete the desired number of reps, repeat the process on your left side.

BRAD'S TRAINING TIPS

- Don't let your upper arm sag as you lift—this reduces the effects of gravity and thus diminishes tension to the target muscles.
- Don't flick your wrist at the top of the movement—this common error fatigues the forearm muscles before sufficiently fatiguing the triceps and reduces the effectiveness of the move.
- Arch your back slightly throughout the movement. Never round your spine—this increases stress on the lumbar area and could lead to injury.

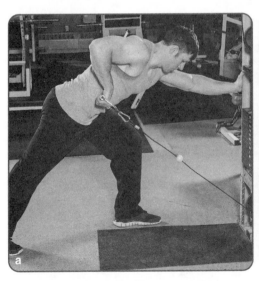
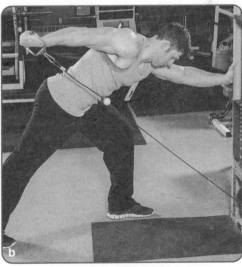

CABLE TRICEPS PRESS-DOWN

TARGET

This move targets the triceps, particularly the middle and lateral heads.

START

With your palms facing each other, grasp the ends of a rope (or loop handles) attached to a high-pulley apparatus. Stand with your feet shoulder-width apart and your torso erect. Slightly bend your knees and hold your core rigid. Bend your elbows to form a 90-degree angle. Press your arms against your sides with your palms facing each other.

MOVEMENT

Keeping your elbows at your sides, straighten your arms as far as comfortably possible. Contract your triceps. Reverse the direction and return to the start position.

BRAD'S TRAINING TIPS

- Don't allow your arms to flare out as you lift—this brings the chest muscles into play at the expense of your triceps.
- Avoid leaning forward for leverage during movement—doing so reduces tension to the target muscles.
- You can perform this move with a variety of attachments, including a curved bar, a straight bar, and loop handles.

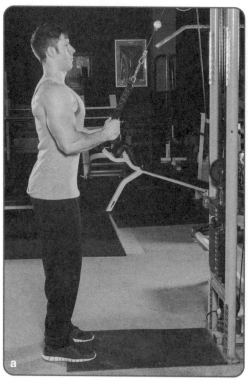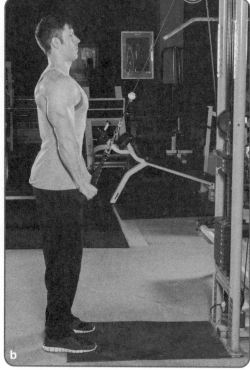

TRICEPS DIP

TARGET

This move targets the triceps.

START

Set up two flat benches several feet apart so that they are parallel with each other. Hold your arms straight and place your palms on the edge of one bench. Place your heels on top of the other bench.

MOVEMENT

Bend your elbows as far as comfortably possible and allow your butt to descend below the level of the bench. Make sure that your elbows stay close to your body throughout the move. Reverse the direction by forcibly straightening your arms and return to the start position.

BRAD'S TRAINING TIPS

- Make the move easier by placing your feet on the floor.
- Increase the intensity of the exercise by placing a weight plate on your lap (variation photo).
- Keep your back close to the bench at all times. If your body gravitates forward, you place increased stress on the shoulder joint.

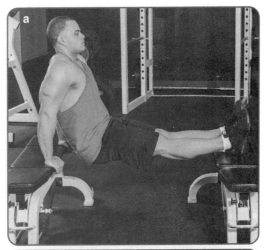

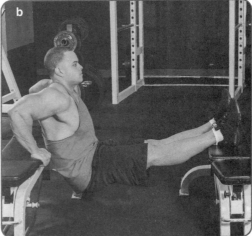

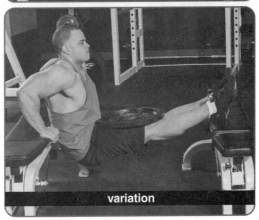

variation

MACHINE TRICEPS DIP

TARGET

This move targets the triceps.

START

Sit upright in the seat of a triceps dip machine and secure your knees firmly under the pads. Grasp the machine handles with your palms facing your sides so that your arms form an angle of approximately 90 degrees.

MOVEMENT

Keeping your torso erect and your elbows in, push the handles down until your arms fully straighten. Contract your triceps. Reverse the direction and return to the start position.

BRAD'S TRAINING TIP

- Keep your upper arms close to your body at all times. Allowing the elbows to flare increases pectoral activation and thereby reduces the work performed by the triceps.

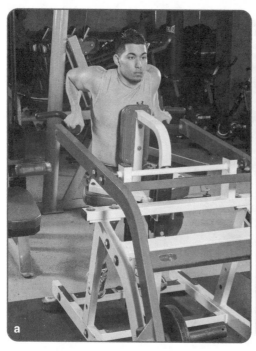
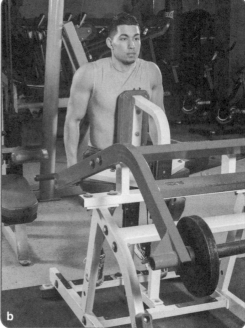

EXERCISES FOR
THE LOWER BODY

This chapter describes and illustrates exercises for the muscles of the lower body: the quadriceps, glutes, hamstrings, and calves. Despite their functional and aesthetic importance, most people seem to train these muscles as an afterthought, performing a few half-hearted sets with minimal effort. Some even neglect working the leg muscles altogether, figuring if they simply wear pants all the time, then no one will notice. Big mistake. Yes, leg training is highly demanding and takes more out of you than any other area of the body. But a muscular lower body with separation between the individual muscles is essential to a balanced, aesthetic physique. There's simply no way around it; after all, you look pretty silly wearing long pants to the beach or a pool party! Bottom line: Train your legs and train them hard!

Read over the descriptions carefully and scrutinize the photos to ensure proper form. I provide training tips for each of these movements to optimize performance. Remember that exercises are merely tools for achieving a means to an end—in this case, muscle development. If an exercise does not feel right to you, simply substitute a comparable move.

WALKING LUNGE

TARGET

This move targets the quads and glutes. Secondary emphasis is placed on the hamstrings.

START

Grasp two dumbbells. Stand in an open area with your feet shoulder-width apart.

MOVEMENT

Take a long stride forward with your right leg and bring your left knee to just above floor level. Then, keeping your shoulders back and your head up throughout the move, step forward with your left leg and allow your right knee to drop down until it is a few inches (about 10 cm) from the floor. Alternate legs and continue for the desired number of reps.

BRAD'S TRAINING TIP

- Don't push forward with your front leg—doing so can place undue stress on the knee. Rather, focus on passively dropping the rear leg so that the front leg forms an approximately 90-degree angle in the finish position.

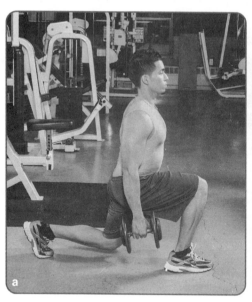
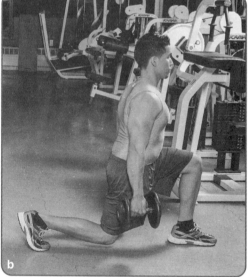

BARBELL LUNGE

TARGET

This move targets the quads and glutes. Secondary emphasis is placed on the hamstrings.

START

Rest a barbell across your shoulders, grasping the bar on both sides to maintain balance. Assume a shoulder-width stance and hold your shoulders back and your chin up.

MOVEMENT

Keeping your core rigid, take a long step forward with your left leg, lowering your body by flexing your left knee and hip in the process. Continue your descent until your right knee is almost in contact with the floor. Reverse the direction by forcibly extending the left hip and knee, bringing the leg backward until you return to the start position. Perform the exercise with your right leg and then alternate legs until you reach the desired number of reps.

BRAD'S TRAINING TIPS

- Make sure your front knee travels in line with the plane of your toes.
- Don't push forward with your front leg—doing so can place undue stress on the knee. Rather, focus on passively dropping the rear leg so that the front leg forms an approximately 90-degree angle in the finish position.

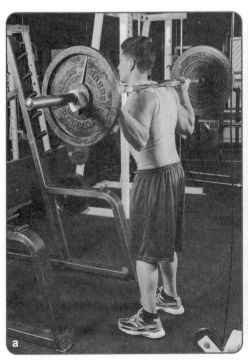
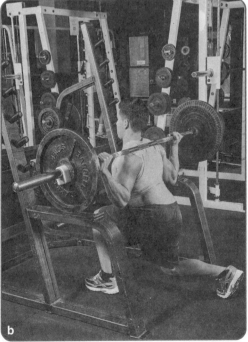

DUMBBELL LUNGE

TARGET

This move targets the quads and glutes. Secondary emphasis is placed on the hamstrings.

START

Grasp two dumbbells and allow them to hang down by your sides, palms facing your body. Assume a shoulder-width stance and hold your shoulders back and your chin up.

MOVEMENT

Keeping your core rigid, take a long step forward with your right leg, lowering your body by flexing your right knee and hip in the process. Continue your descent until your left knee is almost in contact with the floor. Reverse the direction by forcibly extending the right hip and knee, bringing the right leg backward until you return to the start position. Perform the exercise with your left leg and then alternate legs until you reach the desired number of reps.

BRAD'S TRAINING TIPS

- Make sure your front knee travels in line with the plane of your toes.
- Don't push forward with your front leg—doing so can place undue stress on the knee. Rather, focus on passively dropping the rear leg so that the front leg forms an approximately 90-degree angle in the finish position.
- Maintain a forward or slightly upward gaze as you perform the move—this helps prevent rounding at the upper spine.

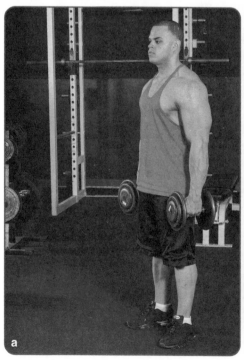
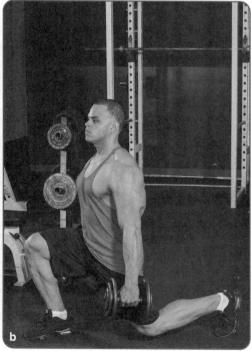

DUMBBELL REVERSE LUNGE

TARGET

This move targets the quads and glutes. Secondary emphasis is placed on the hamstrings.

START

Grasp two dumbbells and allow them to hang down by your sides, palms facing your body. Assume a shoulder-width stance and hold your shoulders back and your chin up.

MOVEMENT

Keeping your core rigid, take a long step backward with your left leg, lowering your body by flexing your right knee and hip in the process. Continue your descent until your left knee is almost in contact with the floor. Reverse the direction by forcibly extending the right hip and knee, bringing your left leg forward until you return to the start position. Repeat the exercise with your right leg and then alternate legs until you reach the desired number of reps.

BRAD'S TRAINING TIPS

- A longer stride emphasizes more of the glutes; a shorter stride targets the quads.
- Maintain a forward or slightly upward gaze as you perform the move—this helps prevent rounding at the upper spine.

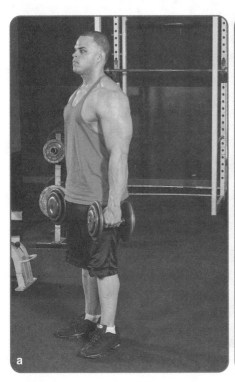
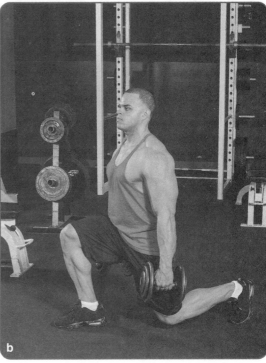

DUMBBELL SIDE LUNGE

TARGET

This move targets the muscles of the lower body, particularly the adductors located along the inner thighs.

START

Assume a relatively wide stance, approximately 1 foot (0.3 m) or more past the width of your shoulders. Grasp two dumbbells and hold them at your sides.

MOVEMENT

Keeping your left leg straight, bend your right knee out to the side until your right thigh is parallel with the floor. Forcefully rise back up and immediately repeat the exercise to your left. Alternate legs until you reach the desired number of reps.

BRAD'S TRAINING TIPS

- Make sure your front knee travels in line with the plane of your toes.
- Maintain a forward or slightly upward gaze as you perform the move—this helps prevent rounding at the upper spine.

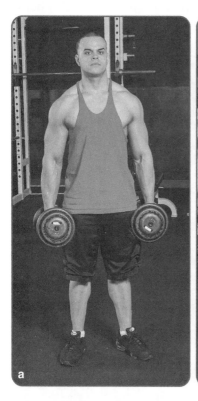

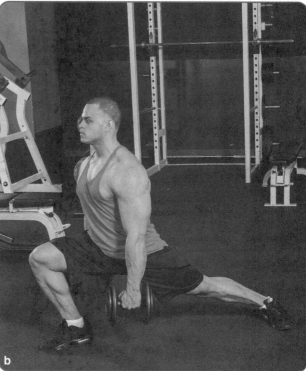

DUMBBELL STEP-UP

TARGET

This move targets the quads and glutes. Secondary emphasis is placed on the hamstrings.

START

Grasp a pair of dumbbells and allow them to hang at your sides. Stand with your feet approximately shoulder-width apart and face the side of a flat bench.

MOVEMENT

Pushing off your left leg, step up on the bench with your right foot and follow with your left foot so that both feet are flat on the bench. Step back down in the reverse order, first with your left foot and then with your right, and return to the start position. Alternate legs for the desired number of reps.

BRAD'S TRAINING TIPS

- A higher step height increases stimulation of the glutes.
- Maintain a forward or slightly upward gaze as you perform the move—this helps prevent rounding at the upper spine.

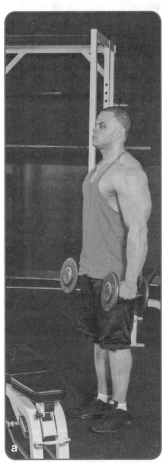
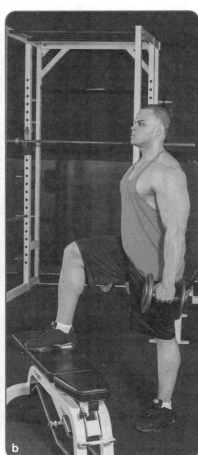
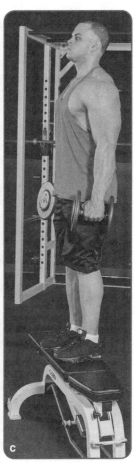

119

BARBELL FRONT SQUAT

TARGET

This move targets the quads and glutes. Secondary emphasis is placed on the hamstrings. Particular emphasis is placed on the muscles of the frontal thighs.

START

Rest a barbell across your upper chest, cross your arms, and hold it in place with both hands. Assume a shoulder-width stance and turn your feet slightly outward. Hold your shoulders back and keep your chin up.

MOVEMENT

Keeping your core rigid, lower your body until your thighs are parallel with the floor. Your lower back should be slightly arched and your heels should stay in contact with the floor at all times. When you reach a "seated" position, reverse the direction by straightening your legs and return to the start position.

BRAD'S TRAINING TIPS

- Your knees should travel in the same plane as your toes at all times.
- Your heels should stay in contact with the floor at all times. If you have trouble keeping your heels down, place a block of wood approximately 1 inch (2.5 cm) thick or a weight plate under them.
- Maintain a forward or slightly upward gaze as you perform the move—this helps prevent rounding at the upper spine.
- Wrap a towel around the bar if it feels uncomfortable on your chest.

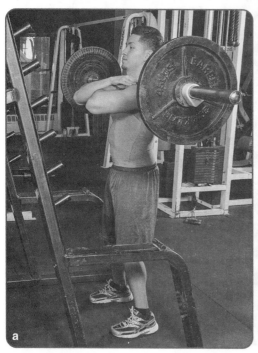
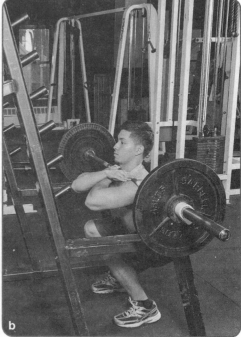

BARBELL BACK SQUAT

TARGET

This move targets the quads and glutes. Secondary emphasis is placed on the hamstrings.

START

Rest a barbell across your shoulders, grasping the bar with both hands. Assume a shoulder-width stance and slightly turn your feet outward.

MOVEMENT

Keeping your core rigid, lower your body until your thighs are parallel with the floor. Your lower back should be slightly arched and your heels should stay in contact with the floor at all times. When you reach a "seated" position, reverse the direction by straightening your legs and return to the start position.

BRAD'S TRAINING TIPS

- Your knees should travel in the same plane as your toes at all times.
- Your heels should stay in contact with the floor at all times. If you have trouble keeping your heels down, place a block of wood approximately 1 inch (2.5 cm) thick or a weight plate under them.
- Maintain a forward or slightly upward gaze as you perform the move—this helps prevent rounding at the upper spine.
- Wrap a towel around the bar if it feels uncomfortable on your neck.

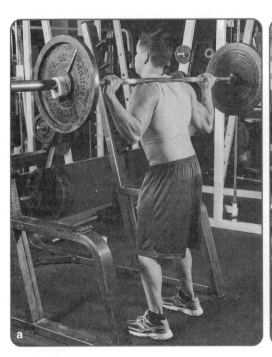
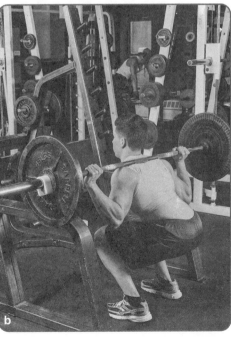

BARBELL SPLIT SQUAT

TARGET

This move targets the quads and glutes. Secondary emphasis is placed on the hamstrings.

START

Rest a barbell across your shoulders, grasping the bar on both sides to maintain balance. Take a long stride forward with your left leg and raise your right heel so that your right foot is on its toes. Hold your shoulders back and your chin up.

MOVEMENT

Keeping your core rigid, lower your body by flexing your left knee and hip. Continue your descent until your right knee is almost in contact with the floor. Reverse the direction by forcibly extending your right hip and knee until you return to the start position. After you complete the desired number of reps, repeat the process with your right leg forward.

BRAD'S TRAINING TIPS

• Make sure your front knee travels in line with the plane of your toes.

• Maintain a forward or slightly upward gaze as you perform the move—this helps prevent rounding at the upper spine.

• Focus on dropping down on your rear leg—this keeps the front knee from pushing too far forward, which can place undue stress on the joint capsule.

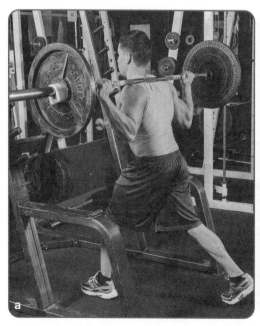
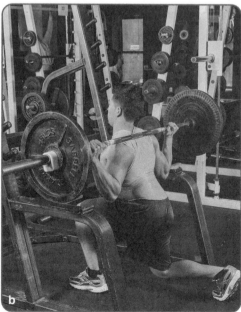

BULGARIAN SQUAT

TARGET

This move targets the quads and glutes. Secondary emphasis is placed on the hamstrings.

START

Grasp two dumbbells and allow your arms to hang down by your sides, palms facing your hips. Stand approximately 2 feet (0.6 m) in front of a raised object (such as a bench or chair) and place your left instep on top of the object. Your back should be straight. Hold your head up and your chest out.

MOVEMENT

Keeping your front foot flat on the floor, lower your body until your right thigh is approximately parallel with the floor. Your lower back should be slightly arched and your right heel should stay in contact with the floor at all times. Reverse the direction by straightening your right leg and returning to the start position. After you complete the desired number of reps, repeat the process on the opposite side.

BRAD'S TRAINING TIPS

- You can increase the difficulty of the exercise by raising the height of the bench.
- Maintain a forward or slightly upward gaze as you perform the move—this helps prevent rounding at the upper spine.

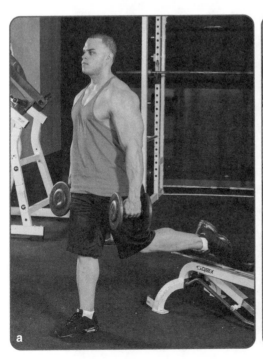
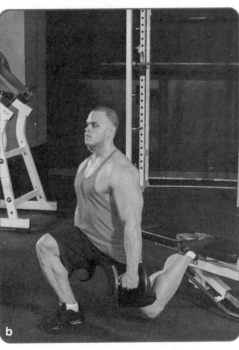

LEG PRESS

TARGET

This move targets the glutes and quads. Secondary emphasis is placed on the hamstrings.

START

Sit back in the seat of an angled leg press machine. Place your feet on the footplate and assume a shoulder-width stance. Keeping your toes angled slightly outward, straighten your legs and unlock the carriage-release bars located on the sides of the machine.

MOVEMENT

Keeping your back pressed firmly against the padded seat, lower your legs and bring your knees in toward your chest. Without bouncing at the bottom of the movement, press the weight up in a controlled fashion and contract your quads. Stop just before locking your knees.

BRAD'S TRAINING TIP

• Placing your feet high on the footplate increases stimulation of the glutes; placing your feet low emphasizes the quads.

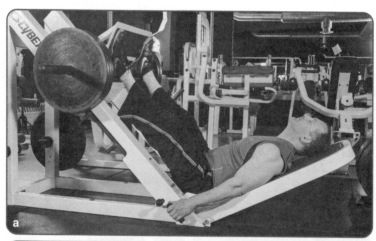

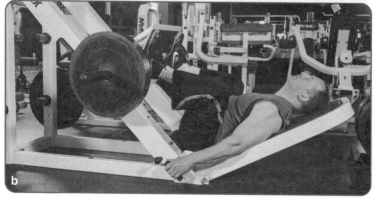

DEADLIFT

TARGET

This moves targets the entire lower-body musculature. It also involves a considerable contribution from many upper-body muscles.

START

Assume a shoulder-width stance a few inches (12-15 cm) in front of a barbell that rests on the floor. Bend your knees and, placing your hands just outside of your legs, grasp the bar with an alternating grip (one hand over the bar, the other hand under the bar). Keep your spine neutral.

MOVEMENT

Keeping your head up, chest out, and arms straight, drive the weight up by forcefully extending your legs and hips. Contract your glutes as you reach the top of the lift and then return to the start position.

BRAD'S TRAINING TIPS

- Keep your shins as close to the bar as possible when you lift—this maximizes leverage in the movement.
- Don't hyperextend your lower back at the top of the lift. Rather, your body should form a straight line as you contract your glutes.
- Use lifting straps if you have trouble holding the weight.

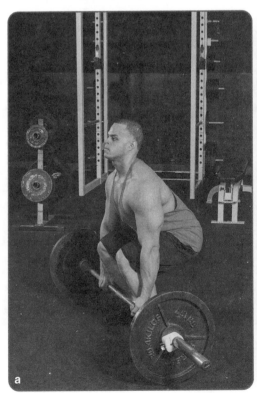
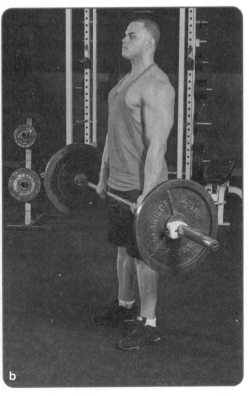

BARBELL HIP THRUST

TARGET

This move targets the glutes. Secondary emphasis is placed on the hamstrings.

START

Sit on the ground with your legs straight, and place your upper back against a secured and padded bench (or step, box, etc.). Position a barbell over your lower legs and roll the bar over the thighs so that it is situated at the crease of your hips slightly above the pelvis. Bend your knees to a 90-degree angle and keep your feet shoulder-width apart and planted firmly on the floor.

MOVEMENT

Keeping your core braced and your spine in a neutral position, raise the barbell off the ground by powerfully contracting your hip extensors until your torso is parallel with the ground. Squeeze your glutes for one count at the top of the movement and then return to the start position.

BRAD'S TRAINING TIPS

- The knees should track directly over the toes and not cave inward.
- Focus on pushing through the entire foot while keeping the soles of your feet flat on the ground.
- Place a pad on the bar to reduce pressure on the lower abdominal region.

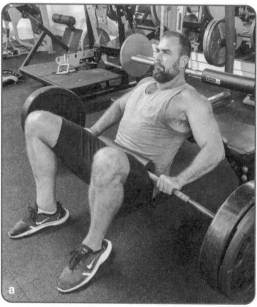
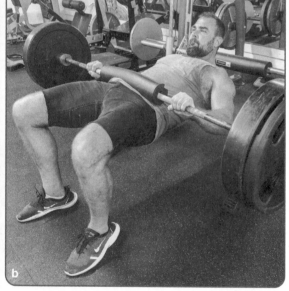

Courtesy of Bret Contreras.

GOOD MORNING

TARGET

This move targets the glutes and hamstrings.

START

Rest a barbell across the tops of your shoulders, grasping the bar on both sides to maintain balance. Assume a shoulder-width stance. Hold your head up and keep your knees and back straight.

MOVEMENT

Keeping your lower back rigid throughout the movement, bend forward at the hips until your upper body is roughly parallel with the floor. In a controlled fashion, reverse the direction and contract your glutes as you rise up along the same path back to the start position.

BRAD'S TRAINING TIPS

- Wrap a towel around the bar if it feels uncomfortable on your neck.
- Move only at the hips, not the waist. Any spinal movement places the vertebrae at increased risk of injury.
- The long moment arm (the distance between the resistance and the axis of rotation) in this exercise makes a rigid core critical.
- This move is not recommended for those with an existing lower-back injury.

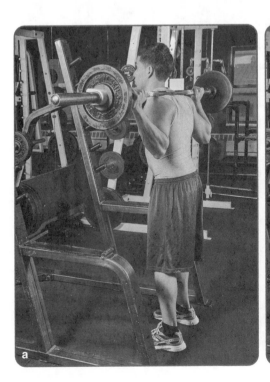
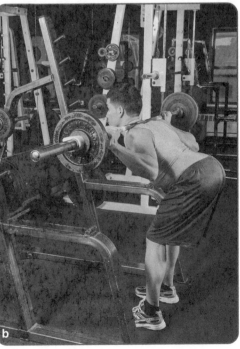

SISSY SQUAT

TARGET

This move targets the quads, particularly the rectus femoris.

START

Assume a shoulder-width stance. Grasp a stationary object with one hand and rise up onto your toes.

MOVEMENT

In one motion, slant your torso back, bend your knees, and lower your body. Thrust your knees forward as you descend and lean back until your torso is as close to parallel with the floor as possible. Then reverse the direction and rise up until you reach the start position.

BRAD'S TRAINING TIPS

- Make sure you remain on your toes throughout the move—keeping your feet planted can result in injury to the knees.
- If the exercise becomes too easy and you are not challenged within the target rep range, you can hold a dumbbell or weight plate to your chest for added resistance.
- This move is generally contraindicated for those with an existing knee injury. When in doubt, check with your physician or physical therapist.

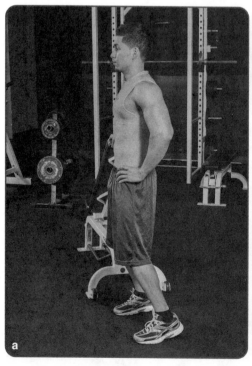
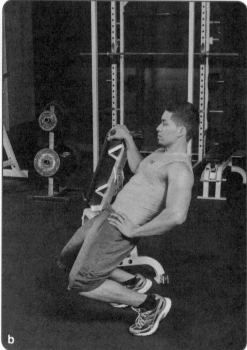

BARBELL STIFF-LEGGED DEADLIFT

TARGET

This move targets the glutes and hamstrings.

START

Stand with your feet about shoulder-width apart, your knees straight and your core rigid. Grasp a barbell and let it hang in front of your body.

MOVEMENT

Keeping your knees straight and your core rigid, bend forward at the hips and lower the barbell until you feel an intense stretch in your hamstrings. Then reverse the direction and contract your glutes as you rise up to the start position.

BRAD'S TRAINING TIPS

- Bend forward only at the hips, not the lower back. The action is purely hip extension, and any spinal movement places the vertebrae at an increased risk of injury.
- Standing on a box, which many people do, is necessary only if you can touch your toes without flexing your spine—a feat few people are able to do.

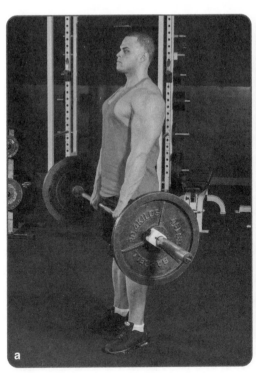
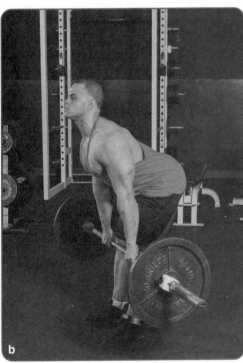

DUMBBELL STIFF-LEGGED DEADLIFT

TARGET

This move targets the glutes and hamstrings.

START

Stand with your feet about shoulder-width apart, your knees straight and your core rigid. Grasp a pair of dumbbells and let them hang in front of your body.

MOVEMENT

Keeping your knees straight and your core rigid, bend forward at the hips and lower the dumbbells until you feel an intense stretch in your hamstrings. Then reverse the direction and forcefully contract your glutes as you rise up to the start position.

BRAD'S TRAINING TIPS

- Bend forward only at the hips, not the lower back. The action is purely hip extension, and any spinal movement places the vertebrae at increased risk of injury.
- Standing on a box, which many people do, is necessary only if you can touch your toes without flexing your spine—a feat few people are able to do.

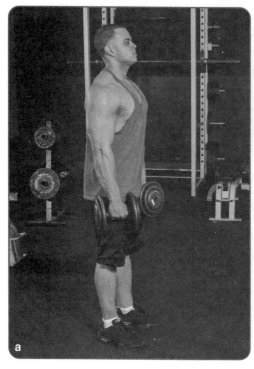
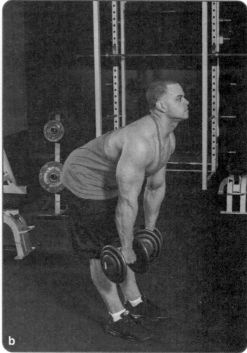

CABLE GLUTE KICKBACK

TARGET

This move targets the glutes, particularly the gluteus maximus, and hamstrings.

START

Attach a cuff to a low-pulley apparatus and secure the cuff to your right ankle. Face the machine and grasp a sturdy object for support.

MOVEMENT

Keeping your upper body motionless and your right leg straight, bring your right foot back as far as comfortably possible. Contract your glutes and return to the start position. After you complete the desired number of reps on your right side, repeat with your left leg.

BRAD'S TRAINING TIP

- To increase activation of the glutes, bend the working knee slightly while performing the move because this decreases activation of the hamstrings.

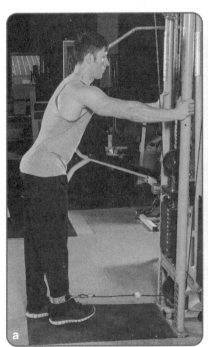
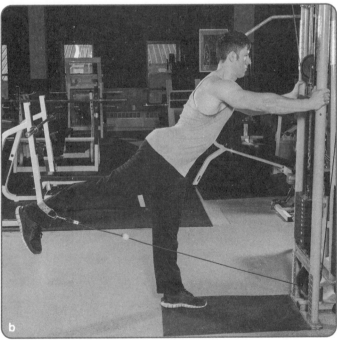

HYPEREXTENSION

TARGET

This move targets the glutes and hamstrings.

START

Lie facedown on a Roman chair. Hook your feet securely under the roller pads and rest your pelvis on the bench pad. Cross your arms over your chest.

MOVEMENT

Keeping your lower body rigid and your head neutral or tilted slightly upward, lift your chest and shoulders up until your body is in a straight line. Contract your glutes and return along the same path to the start position.

BRAD'S TRAINING TIPS

- Don't move your head during the movement—doing so can strain the neck muscles.
- Don't hyperextend your lower back—this can cause lumbar injury.
- To increase the level of difficulty, hold a weight plate or medicine ball against your chest as you perform the move.

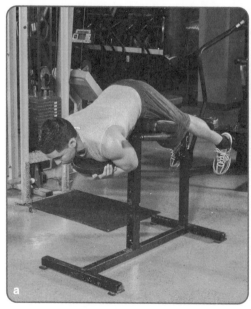 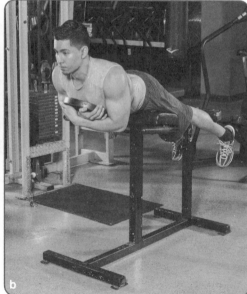

REVERSE HYPEREXTENSION

TARGET

This move targets the glutes and hamstrings.

START

Lie facedown on a Roman chair and grasp the metal post under the roller pads. Rest your chest and abdomen on the bench pad. Your legs should hang down as far as possible without touching the floor.

MOVEMENT

Lift your legs up until your ankles and the back of your head are in a straight line. Contract your glutes and return along the same path back to the start position.

BRAD'S TRAINING TIPS

- Your knees should remain rigid throughout the move. Don't use momentum by flexing and then whipping the lower legs straight.
- Don't hyperextend the lower back—this can cause lumbar injury.
- If the move becomes too easy, attach leg weights to your ankles.

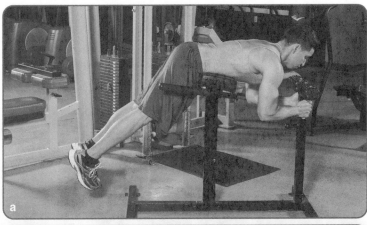

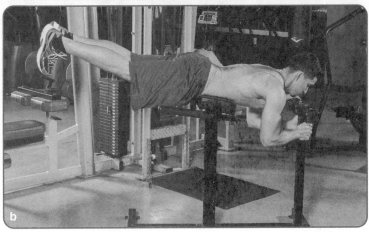

133

LEG EXTENSION

TARGET

This move targets the quads.

START

Sit upright in a leg extension machine so that the undersides of your knees touch the edge of the seat. Bend your knees and place your insteps under the roller pad located at the bottom of the machine. Grasp the machine's handles for support, stiffen your core, and straighten your back.

MOVEMENT

Keeping your thighs and your upper body immobile, lift your feet up until your legs are almost parallel with the floor. Contract your quads and then reverse the direction and return to the start position.

BRAD'S TRAINING TIPS

- Because of the high shear forces associated with this move, it may be contraindicated for those with knee problems. When in doubt, check with your physician or physical therapist.
- Turning your feet in or out offers no added benefit and can place the knee joint in a compromised position. Keep them pointed straight ahead.
- Don't allow the moving weight stack to touch the nonmoving part of the weight stack at the completion of a repetition—doing so takes tension off the quads.

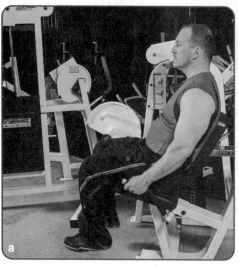 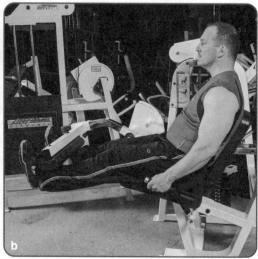

UNILATERAL LEG EXTENSION

TARGET

This move targets the quads.

START

Sit upright in a leg extension machine so that the undersides of your knees touch the edge of the seat. Bend your right knee and place your right instep under the roller pad located at the bottom of the machine. Keep your left leg back so that it is off the roller pad. Grasp the machine's handles for support, stiffen your core, and straighten your back.

MOVEMENT

Keeping your thighs and your upper body immobile, lift your right foot up until your right lower leg is almost parallel with the floor. Contract your quads and then reverse the direction and return to the start position. After you complete the desired number of reps, repeat the process on your left side.

BRAD'S TRAINING TIPS

- Because of the high shear forces associated with this move, it may be contraindicated for those with knee problems. When in doubt, check with your physician or physical therapist.
- Turning your feet in or out offers no added benefit and can place the knee joint in a compromised position. Keep them pointed straight ahead.
- Don't allow the moving weight stack to touch the nonmoving part of the weight stack at the completion of a repetition—doing so takes tension off the quads.

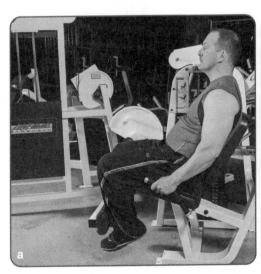 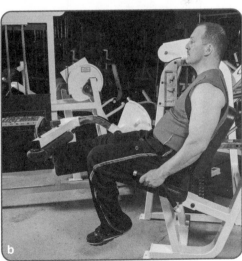

LYING LEG CURL

TARGET

This move targets the hamstrings.

START

Lie facedown on a lying leg curl machine. Hook your heels under the roller pad. Grasp the handles (if available) or the bench pad for stability.

MOVEMENT

Keeping your thighs pressed against the bench surface, bend your knees and bring your feet up and toward your body, stopping just short of touching your feet to your butt or as close to that point as is comfortably possible. Contract your hamstrings and then reverse the direction and return to the start position.

BRAD'S TRAINING TIPS

- Don't allow the moving weight stack to touch the nonmoving part of the weight stack at the completion of a repetition—doing so takes tension off the hamstrings.
- To increase hamstrings involvement, keep your calves plantarflexed throughout the movement, which reduces activation of the gastrocnemii.

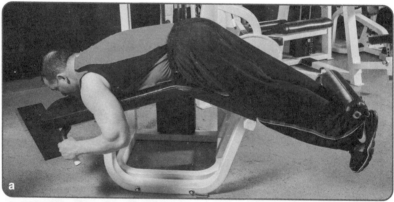

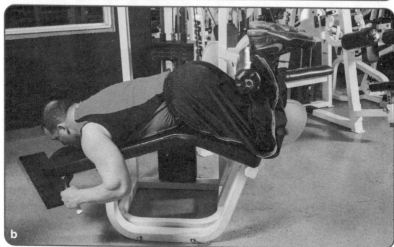

MACHINE KNEELING LEG CURL

TARGET

This move targets the hamstrings.

START

Place your left knee on the knee pad of a kneeling leg curl machine and hook your right heel under the roller pad. Place your forearms on the restraint pad for support. Keep your back flat and your torso immobile throughout the move.

MOVEMENT

Bring your right foot up and toward your body, stopping just short of touching your foot to your butt or as close to that point as is comfortably possible. Contract your right hamstrings and then reverse the direction and return to the start position. After you complete the desired number of reps, repeat the process on your left side.

BRAD'S TRAINING TIPS

- Don't allow the moving weight stack to touch the nonmoving part of the weight stack at the start position of the move—doing so takes tension off the hamstrings.
- To increase hamstrings involvement, keep your calves plantarflexed throughout the movement, which reduces activation of the gastrocnemii.

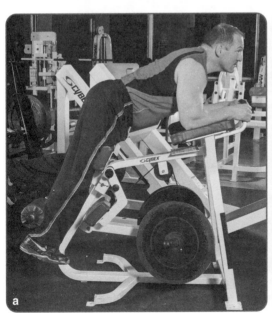
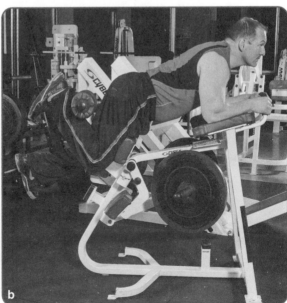

MACHINE SEATED LEG CURL

TARGET

This move targets the hamstrings.

START

Sit in a seated leg curl machine. Keep your back flat against the back rest and place your heels over the roller pads. Lower the leg restraint over your thighs.

MOVEMENT

Press your feet downward as far as comfortably possible. Contract your hamstrings when your knees are fully bent. Then reverse the direction and return to the start position.

BRAD'S TRAINING TIPS

- Don't allow the moving weight stack to touch the nonmoving part of the weight stack at the start position of the move—doing so takes tension off the hamstrings.
- To increase hamstrings involvement, keep your calves plantarflexed throughout the movement, which reduces activation of the gastrocnemii.

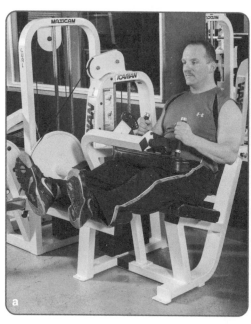 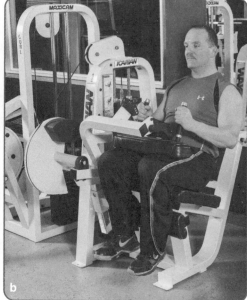

TOE PRESS

TARGET

This move targets the calf muscles, particularly the gastrocnemius.

START

Sit upright in a leg press machine and press your back firmly against the padded seat. Place the balls of your feet a comfortable distance apart on the bottom of the footplate, keeping your heels off the footplate. Straighten your legs, unlock the carriage-release bars, and drop your heels below your toes as far as comfortably possible.

MOVEMENT

Keeping your knees immobile, press your toes as high up as you can until your ankles are fully extended. Contract your calves and then reverse the direction and return to the start position.

BRAD'S TRAINING TIPS

- Never bounce during the stretched position of the move—this increases the risk of injury to the Achilles tendon.
- Turning your toes outward can place increased emphasis on the medial head of the gastrocnemius; turning your toes inward can help target the lateral head of the gastrocnemius.

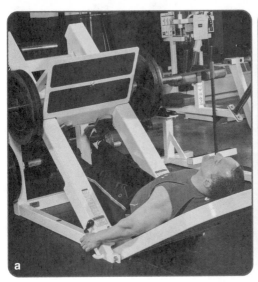 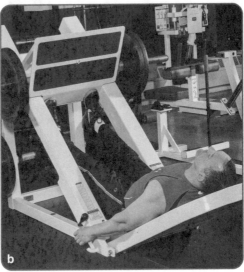

MACHINE SEATED CALF RAISE

TARGET

This move targets the calves, particularly the soleus muscle.

START

Sit in a seated calf machine and place the restraint pad tightly across your thighs. Place the balls of your feet on the footplate and drop your heels below your toes as far as comfortably possible.

MOVEMENT

Rise as high as you can on your toes until your ankles are fully extended. Contract your calves and then reverse the direction and return to the start position.

BRAD'S TRAINING TIPS

- Never bounce during the stretched position of the move—this increases the risk of injury to the Achilles tendon.
- Because the gastrocnemius muscle is not very active in this exercise, it is best to keep your toes pointed straight ahead.

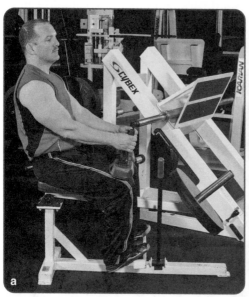 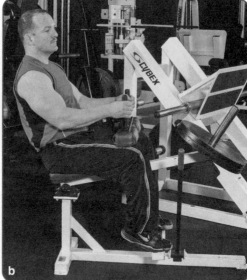

MACHINE STANDING CALF RAISE

TARGET

This move targets the calf muscles, particularly the gastrocnemius.

START

Place your shoulders under the restraint pad of a standing calf machine. Place the balls of your feet on the footplate and drop your heels below your toes as far as comfortably possible.

MOVEMENT

Rise as high as you can on your toes until your ankles are fully extended. Contract your calves and then reverse the direction and return to the start position.

BRAD'S TRAINING TIPS

- Never bounce during the stretched position of the move—this increases the risk of injury to the Achilles tendon.
- Turning your toes outward can place an increased emphasis on the medial head of the gastrocnemius; turning your toes inward can help to target the lateral head of the gastrocnemius.

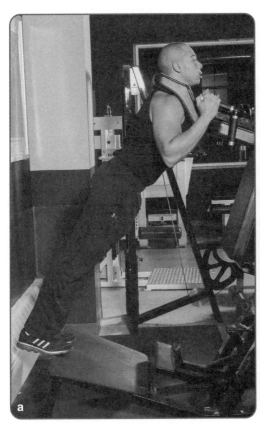 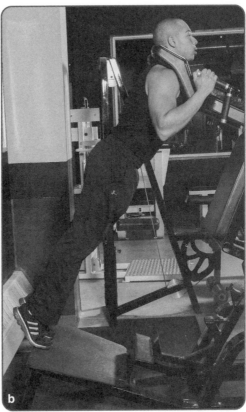

141

CHAPTER 6

M.A.X. WARM-UP

A pre-workout warm-up can help to prepare your body for the demands of intense exercise. The warm-up contains two basic components: a general warm-up and a specific warm-up. Here's what you need to know about each component for a safe, effective workout.

GENERAL WARM-UP

The general warm-up consists of a brief bout of low-intensity, large-muscle group, aerobic exercise. The objective is to elevate your core temperature and increase blood flow, which in turn enhances the speed of nerve impulses, increases nutrient delivery to working muscles and the removal of metabolic by-products, and facilitates oxygen release from hemoglobin and myoglobin.

A direct correlation exists between muscle temperature and exercise performance: When a muscle is warm, it has a greater capacity to contract. As a rule, the higher a muscle's temperature (within a safe physiological range), the better its contractility. And because better contractility translates into greater force production, you'll achieve higher levels of mechanical tension during your training, conceivably helping to enhance muscle development.

What's more, an elevated core temperature diminishes a joint's resistance to flow (viscosity). This is accomplished via the uptake of synovial fluid, which is secreted from the synovial membrane to lubricate the joint. The net effect is an increase in range of motion and improved joint-related resiliency. Better yet, these factors combine to reduce the risk of a training-related injury.

Suffice to say, there's a potential benefit to including a general warm-up prior to each workout.

Virtually any cardiorespiratory activity can be used for the general warm-up. Exercises on equipment such as stationary bikes, stair climbers, and treadmills are viable options, as are most calisthenic-type exercises (e.g., jumping jacks, burpees). Choose whatever activity you desire as long as the basic objective is met.

The intensity for the general warm-up should be low. To estimate intensity of training, I recommend using a rating of perceived exertion (RPE) scale. My preference is the category-ratio RPE scale, which grades perceived effort on a scale from 1 to 10 (see table 6.1), because it is more intuitive than the original

Table 6.1   10-Point Category-Ratio RPE
Scale

RPE	INTENSITY
1	No exertion at all
2	Extremely light
3	Very light
4	Somewhat light
5	Light
6	Somewhat hard
7	Hard
8	Very hard
9	Extremely hard
10	Maximal exertion

RPE scale proposed by Swedish researcher Gunnar Borg. Aim for an RPE of around 5 or so, which for most people is a moderate-paced walk or slow jog. You also can use the talk test as an intensity gauge. With this method, you assess intensity based on your ability to carry on a conversation; if you have to pause to take a breath while speaking a sentence, you're working too hard.

Five to 10 minutes is all you need for the general warm-up—just enough to break a light sweat. Your resources should not be taxed, nor should you feel fatigued or out of breath during or after performance. If so, you're training too hard and should decrease the exercise intensity. Remember, this is not intended to be a cardio session. The goal here is merely to warm your body tissues and accelerate blood flow, not to achieve cardiorespiratory benefits or reduce body fat.

SPECIFIC WARM-UP

The specific warm-up can be considered an extension of the general warm-up. By using exercises that are similar to the activities in the workout, the specific warm-up enhances neuromuscular efficiency for the exercise you are about to perform. In essence, your body gets to rehearse the movements before you perform them at a high level of intensity, translating into better performance during your working sets.

To optimize transfer of training, the exercises in the specific warm-up should mimic the movements in the workout as closely as possible. For example, if you are going to perform a bench press, the specific warm-up should ideally include light sets of the bench press. A viable alternative would be to perform push-ups because the movement pattern is similar to that of a bench press, although the specificity, and thus transfer, would not be as great as with light sets of the given movement. Always stop specific warm-up sets well short of failure. The objective is not to fatigue your muscles but rather to get a feel for the exercise so that you're physically and mentally prepared for intense training.

The specific warm-up is particularly important when training in low rep ranges, as will be the case in the M.A.X. strength phase. I recommend at least a couple of specific warm-up sets per exercise during low-rep training. As a general rule, the first set should be performed at approximately 40-50% of the 1RM and the second set at approximately 60-70% of the 1RM. The reps in reserve (RIR) should be at least a four in these sets—any higher is superfluous and potentially counterproductive because it will cause undue fatigue. Following the specific warm-up, you should be ready and able to plow into your working sets.

The need for specific warm-up sets when training in medium to high rep ranges remains questionable. I previously collaborated on a study that investigated the effects of a warm-up on the ability to carry out repetitions to failure at 80% of the 1RM (a weight that allows performance of about eight reps) in the squat, bench press, and arm curl (3). The verdict: Warming up showed no beneficial effects on the number of repetitions performed in medium to high rep-range training, nor in a measure called the fatigue index, which is a formula that assesses the decline in the number of repetitions across the first and last sets of each exercise.

At face value these results suggest that warming up is pretty much useless prior to submaximal resistance training. Despite the currently held belief that a specific warm-up enhances exercise performance, no benefits were seen when compared to no warm-up at all. Intuitively, this seems to make sense, given that the initial repetitions of submaximal lifts are in effect their own specific warm-up, and increasing core temperature might be superfluous from a performance standpoint when multiple reps are performed.

It should be noted, however, that we found a slight advantage to performing a specific warm-up prior to the squat (although results did not rise to statistical significance); alternatively, the specific warm-up prior to the arm curl seemed to be somewhat detrimental. Thus, more complex movement patterns appear to benefit from the practice effect of a specific warm-up; on the other hand, it's seemingly of little value prior to more simple exercises.

Taking the evidence into account, here's my recommendation: When performing medium rep-range work (8-12 reps per set), perform a specific warm-up prior to multi-joint free weight exercises. One set at about 50% of the 1RM at an RIR of ≥4 is all you need to obtain any potential benefits; there's no need for warm-ups on single-joint movements.

Specific warm-up sets are not necessary when training with high reps (15+ reps per set). In this instance, you're already using relatively light weights, and the initial repetitions of each working set therefore serve as rehearsal reps. What's more, performance of warm-up sets during high-rep training blocks is counterproductive to the goal of maximizing training density to bring about desired metabolic adaptations.

WHAT ABOUT STRETCHING?

Static stretching is commonly included as part of a pre-lifting warm-up. This method of flexibility training involves moving a joint through its range of motion to the point where you feel slight discomfort, and then holding the position for a period of time (generally about 30 seconds). Most protocols involve performing several sets of static holds and then moving on to stretches for other muscles. It's commonly believed that the addition of stretching exercises to a warm-up further reduces injury risk while enhancing physical performance.

In recent years, however, the benefits of pre-exercise static stretching have come under scrutiny. A large body of research shows that the practice does not decrease injury risk (5). Yes, improving flexibility can conceivably help in injury prevention. Tight muscles have been implicated as a cause of training-related injury, and improving flexibility can reduce this possibility. Because stretching exercises improve range of motion, including them as a component of an exercise program may potentially enhance overall workout safety. However, the benefits are not specific to stretching prior to training. All that matters is achieving adequate range of motion to properly carry out exercise performance.

The most important consideration here is to make sure your muscles are warm before performing static stretches. This reduces joint viscosity, ensuring that muscles and connective tissues are sufficiently prepped to endure passive or active lengthening.

So you might be thinking: Why not include some basic stretches after the general warm-up? After all, your core temperature is elevated and joint viscosity is reduced. What's the harm, right?

Interestingly, some evidence shows that static stretching performed before a workout can have a detrimental impact on exercise performance (4). This is most applicable to activities requiring high force output, such as heavy resistance training. The primary theory proposed to account for these performance decrements is a decrease in musculotendinous stiffness. The musculotendinous unit (the muscle and its associated tendons) is responsible for generating the force to carry out movement. The musculotendinous unit has increased laxity following stretching, which in turn impairs force transmission, like an overstretched rubber band. The upshot is a reduced capacity to lift a given load.

However, caution needs to be used when extrapolating this research to a lifting session. First, most of the studies in question used excessive stretching protocols—in some cases upward of 30 minutes stretching a single joint! Most pre-workout stretching routines involve only a minute or two per joint, and it's highly questionable whether such brief stretching bouts have any performance-related detriments. Moreover, the vast majority of research on the topic is specific to strength- and power-related activities. Whether negative effects of stretching on performance are seen when training with medium- to high-rep schemes remains speculative.

Given the uncertainty of evidence, you're best off performing static stretches immediately after your workout (assuming increased flexibility is desired). Your body is already warm from engaging in intense exercise, and it generally feels good to cool down by elongating muscles that have been repeatedly contracted. Some research even shows that post-workout stretching may alleviate delayed-onset muscle soreness (see the sidebar, What Causes Muscle Soreness After a Workout?, in this chapter), although the extent of the reduction probably isn't all that meaningful (1).

WHAT CAUSES MUSCLE SORENESS AFTER A WORKOUT?

Following an intense workout, many people feel sore in their trained muscles. This phenomenon, called delayed-onset muscle soreness (DOMS), generally develops a day or two after training and can last 72 hours or more. The soreness can be mild or very severe, depending on a number of factors including genetics, muscle action, and intensity of effort, among others.

The cause of DOMS is often misunderstood. Contrary to popular belief, it's totally unrelated to a buildup of lactic acid. The truth is, lactate is rapidly cleared from muscles following a workout. Within an hour or two post-exercise, it's either completely oxidized or used for glycogen resynthesis. Because DOMS doesn't manifest until at least 24 hours after a training session, it therefore follows that lactic acid cannot play a part in its origin.

So, what causes DOMS? It's actually a product of damage to muscle tissue. Intense exercise produces small microtears in the working muscle fibers, primarily as a result of eccentric activity (i.e., lengthening a muscle against tension). These microtears allow calcium to escape from the muscles, disrupting their intracellular balance. Metabolic by-products are subsequently produced, which in turn interact with the free nerve endings surrounding the damaged fibers, resulting in localized pain and stiffness.

In response, white blood cells migrate to the site of injury, generating free radicals that further exacerbate the sensation of pain. The discomfort can last for several days or even up to a week, depending on the extent of muscle damage.

So don't blame lactic acid buildup for making you sore after a workout. It's merely a sign that you've worked the fibers in an unaccustomed fashion. If you experience DOMS, the best thing you can do is stay active in the post-exercise period, thereby enhancing blood flow to the affected area. This will expedite the delivery of nutrients to the muscles, accelerating the rate of their repair and reducing the associated discomfort. Other remedies such as stretching, foam rolling, heat packs, and massage have been proposed as therapies, although supporting evidence of their effectiveness remains largely uncertain. That said, since the only overt downside to these remedies is the investment of time, feel free to give them a try.

If you want to include some flexibility work prior to lifting, consider dynamic stretches: slow, controlled movements taken through their full range of motion. Examples are arm swings, shoulder circles, high steps, and hip twists. Choose dynamic stretches that are specific to the joint actions being trained in your workout. Perform several sets for each dynamic stretch, attempting to move the body segment farther and farther in a comfortable range with each set.

Contrary to popular belief, you don't necessarily have to include a stretching component in your regular routine. Increased flexibility results in decreased joint stability. Being too flexible, therefore, actually increases injury risk. Thus, stretch only those joints that are tight, and avoid any additional specific flexibility-oriented exercise for joints that already have adequate range of motion to carry out your required activities of daily living.

Moreover, it's important to note that resistance training in itself actually improves flexibility. Provided that you train through a complete range of motion, multi-set lifting protocols produce similar increases in flexibility to those seen with static stretching routines, at least during the early stages of training (2). In essence, resistance training serves as an active form of flexibility training whereby a muscle is contracted and then immediately lengthened. When performed on a regular basis, it can keep you mobile and limber. We can therefore put to rest the myth that lifting binds you up!

M.A.X.
BREAK-IN ROUTINE

Make no mistake: The M.A.X. Muscle Plan is a hard-core muscle-building routine. As such, it's intended for those who have at least some lifting experience, ideally six months or more. If you lack the requisite experience, the program is likely to overwhelm your recuperative abilities and lead to an overtrained state.

If you're relatively new to resistance training or perhaps coming back from a prolonged layoff from lifting, don't worry. I created the break-in routine with you in mind. It's a conditioning routine that is designed to prepare your body to deal with the rigorous nature of the M.A.X. Muscle Plan.

If you're a seasoned, active lifter, feel free to skip this chapter and proceed to the strength phase of the program. Before doing so, however, be sure to honestly assess your ability to handle intensive exercise. Should you attempt the program before you're ready, you're bound to become overtrained. This will set your progress back potentially weeks if not months. If you have any doubt about whether you're prepared for the program, err on the side of caution and start with the break-in routine. Better safe than sorry.

PROGRAM PROTOCOL

The break-in routine is a total-body workout in which you train all the major muscles during each session. It's an eight-week mesocycle and consists of two training blocks. Each block includes four one-week microcycles.

Block 1 is an initial break-in routine. It's for those who have no experience whatsoever or who are coming back after a long layoff from lifting. During this block, multi-joint movements are incorporated whenever possible, with the exception of exercises for the arms and calves. Exercise selection is very limited, and you'll perform the same basic movements during each session. While this might seem rudimentary and a tad boring, it's an important conditioning strategy. The primary adaptations during the early stages of training involve your nervous system; muscle hypertrophy is almost nonexistent for the first month or so. During the early stages of training, your body gets used to new movement patterns and finds the most economical way to perform a given exercise. Focusing on a limited number of movements facilitates skill acquisition and allows coordinated motor programs to develop.

You'll train exclusively with relatively high repetitions (15-20 per set) during this block. The higher rep range affords more practice and helps ingrain movement patterns into your subconscious mind. Moreover, it takes the onus away from generating high amounts of force and allows you to concentrate on proper technique. Remember, your sole objective is to get a feel for exercise performance. Once you learn the basic movements and commit their execution to your subconscious, muscle development will follow.

Block 2 is an extended break-in routine that builds on the skills you acquired during the initial break-in routine. At this point you'll have developed basic neuromuscular coordination and solidified technique in fundamental movement patterns. During block 2 you'll expand your ability to perform these movement patterns with a greater variety of exercises and varying levels of intensity. To accomplish this task, you'll follow a fairly traditional undulating periodization schedule that rotates between light, medium, and heavy weeks. You'll use a combination of single- and multi-joint movements that change throughout the week. Sets will require increasingly greater levels of effort, and you'll take the final set to the point of momentary muscle failure.

Throughout the break-in phase, perform repetitions in a deliberate, controlled fashion. Aim to develop a strong mind–muscle connection. The sooner you are able to mentally focus on making the target muscle do the majority of the work, the more quickly you'll make progress. Importantly, avoid speeding up tempo simply to complete a set. This will only cause you to develop bad habits that can be difficult to rectify in the future.

PROGRAM SPECIFICS

As noted, the break-in phase comprises two training blocks. Here are the particulars of each block.

BLOCK 1

Block 1 is the initial break-in routine. It comprises four one-week microcycles. During the first three microcycles, you'll work out on three nonconsecutive days per week (e.g., Monday, Wednesday, and Friday) and train all the major muscle groups during each session. One exercise will be performed per muscle group. You'll perform three sets per exercise and take approximately two minutes of rest between sets. The loading zone for all four microcycles should correspond to 15-20 reps per set. Gradually increase effort on a weekly basis over the first three microcycles as follows.

During the first microcycle in block 1 (week 1 of the mesocycle), your level of effort on all sets should correspond to reps in reserve (RIR) of approximately 4, meaning that the lifts are relatively easy but pose a slight challenge (i.e., you'll have about four reps left in the tank). You shouldn't be struggling on any of the lifts. Rather, your goal is simply to get a feel for the movements and develop coordination between the working muscles so that exercises are performed in a smooth, controlled fashion. Rest intervals should last approximately two minutes between sets.

During the second microcycle in block 1 (week 2), your level of effort on all sets should correspond to an RIR of 3. The lifts should begin to get a little more difficult, but not to the extent that you struggle on the last rep. Concentrate on honing your form to further develop neuromuscular coordination. Rest intervals again should last approximately two minutes between sets.

During the third microcycle in block 1 (week 3), your level of effort on all sets should correspond to an RIR of 1 or 2, meaning that the lifts are quite hard. At this level, the weights should significantly tax your abilities. Avoid training to all-out failure, however, because doing so provides little advantage at this point and may overtax your recuperative abilities. Keep your focus on hardwiring the neural circuitry between your brain and your muscles so that movements become second nature—the sole purpose of this training block. Keep rest intervals at approximately two minutes between sets.

The fourth microcycle in block 1 (week 4) is a deload phase. You'll train two days per week, allowing 72 hours between sessions (e.g., Monday and Thursday or Tuesday and Friday), and follow a total-body routine that works all the major muscle groups during each session. You'll perform one exercise of three sets per muscle group. Loads should equate to 15-20 reps per set, with two-minute rest intervals. Sets should not be overly challenging. Aim for an RIR of 4 or so. If you find the last rep at all difficult to complete, lighten the weight!

By the end of the fourth microcycle, you should be comfortable performing the exercises in good form. If so, progress to block 2. If not, repeat block 1 until you develop the necessary coordination and control for carrying out each movement. When in doubt, repeat the bout; it's always best to err on the side of caution.

BLOCK 2

Block 2 is the extended break-in routine. Similar to block 1, it comprises four one-week microcycles. During the first three microcycles, you'll work out on three nonconsecutive days per week (e.g., Monday, Wednesday, and Friday) and train all the major muscle groups during each session. One exercise will be performed per muscle group. You'll perform three sets per exercise in an undulating-type protocol whereby rep range and rest interval are modified to target specific daily goals. A greater variety of exercises are incorporated into the routine to acclimate your neuromuscular system to different movements. Intensity of effort will increase each week over the course of the first three microcycles, with the last set of each exercise taken to the point of muscle failure (except in the third and fourth microcycles) as follows.

The first microcycle in block 2 (week 5 of the mesocycle) focuses on metabolic conditioning. As such, you'll employ a loading zone corresponding to 15-20 reps per set. Perform the first set at an RIR of about 3, perform the second set at an RIR of about 1 or 2, and take the final set to the point of concentric muscle failure. Rest intervals should last approximately 30 seconds between sets.

The second microcycle in block 2 (week 6) targets hypertrophy-type adaptations. You'll employ an 8-10 rep range (except the abs, which are trained with higher repetitions). Perform the first set at an RIR of about 3, perform the second set at an RIR of about 1 or 2, and take the final set to the point of concentric muscle failure. Rest intervals should last approximately two minutes between sets.

The third microcycle in block 2 (week 7) focuses on strength development and thus employs a heavy-load scheme corresponding to three to five reps per set (except the abs, which are trained with higher repetitions). Perform the first set at an RIR of about 3, perform the second set at an RIR of about 2, and take the final set to just short of failure so that you're leaving a rep in the tank (RIR of approximately 1). Rest intervals should last approximately three minutes between sets.

The fourth microcycle in block 2 (week 8) is a deload phase. You'll train two days per week, allowing 72 hours between sessions (e.g., Monday and Thursday), and follow a total-body routine that works all the major muscle groups during each session. You'll perform one exercise of three sets per muscle group using a loading zone of 15-20 reps per set. Sets should not be overly challenging. Aim for an RIR of 4 or so. If you're at all struggling on the last rep, lighten the weight! Rest intervals should last approximately two minutes between sets.

Generally speaking, I recommend that novice exercisers repeat the extended break-in routine several times before initiating the M.A.X. Muscle Plan. This helps ensure that you're fully prepared for the intense stresses of the training program and diminishes the potential for becoming overtrained. That said, progress is always specific to the individual. Thus, gauge your preparedness at the end of the mesocycle and decide whether you're ready to move forward.

Table 7.1 summarizes the break-in protocol, and sample routines (tables 7.2 through 7.9) are provided on the subsequent pages. These routines should serve as a basic template for constructing your workouts. Modify specific exercises and other training variables according to your individual needs and abilities.

Table 7.1   Summary of Break-In Protocol

TRAINING VARIABLE	PROTOCOL
Repetitions	3-20
Sets	3 per exercise
Rest interval	30 sec to 3 min
Tempo	Mind–muscle connection
Frequency	3 days per week
Effort	0-4 RIR

Table 7.2   Break-In Week 1: Block 1 Microcycle 1

Perform these exercises at an RIR of approximately 4.

DAY	TARGET MUSCLES	EXERCISES	PAGE
Monday	Total body	Dumbbell chest press (3 sets @ 15-20 reps)	53
		Dumbbell one-arm row (3 sets @ 15-20 reps)	35
		Dumbbell shoulder press (3 sets @ 15-20 reps)	81
		Dumbbell standing biceps curl (3 sets @ 15-20 reps)	92
		Cable triceps press-down (3 sets @ 15-20 reps)	110
		Barbell back squat (3 sets @ 15-20 reps)	121
		Lying leg curl (3 sets @ 15-20 reps)	136
		Machine standing calf raise (3 sets @ 15-20 reps)	141
		Crunch (3 sets @ 15-20 reps)	64
Tuesday	Off		
Wednesday	Total body	Dumbbell chest press (3 sets @ 15-20 reps)	53
		Dumbbell one-arm row (3 sets @ 15-20 reps)	35
		Dumbbell shoulder press (3 sets @ 15-20 reps)	81
		Dumbbell standing biceps curl (3 sets @ 15-20 reps)	92
		Cable triceps press-down (3 sets @ 15-20 reps)	110
		Barbell back squat (3 sets @ 15-20 reps)	121
		Lying leg curl (3 sets @ 15-20 reps)	136
		Machine standing calf raise (3 sets @ 15-20 reps)	141
		Crunch (3 sets @ 15-20 reps)	64
Thursday	Off		
Friday	Total body	Dumbbell chest press (3 sets @ 15-20 reps)	53
		Dumbbell one-arm row (3 sets @ 15-20 reps)	35
		Dumbbell shoulder press (3 sets @ 15-20 reps)	81
		Dumbbell standing biceps curl (3 sets @ 15-20 reps)	92
		Cable triceps press-down (3 sets @ 15-20 reps)	110
		Barbell back squat (3 sets @ 15-20 reps)	121
		Lying leg curl (3 sets @ 15-20 reps)	136
		Machine standing calf raise (3 sets @ 15-20 reps)	141
		Crunch (3 sets @ 15-20 reps)	64
Saturday	Off		
Sunday	Off		

Table 7.3   Break-In Week 2: Block 1 Microcycle 2

Perform these exercises at an RIR of 3.

DAY	TARGET MUSCLES	EXERCISES	PAGE
Monday	Total body	Dumbbell chest press (3 sets @ 15-20 reps)	53
		Dumbbell one-arm row (3 sets @ 15-20 reps)	35
		Dumbbell shoulder press (3 sets @ 15-20 reps)	81
		Dumbbell standing biceps curl (3 sets @ 15-20 reps)	92
		Cable triceps press-down (3 sets @ 15-20 reps)	110
		Barbell back squat (3 sets @ 15-20 reps)	121
		Lying leg curl (3 sets @ 15-20 reps)	136
		Machine standing calf raise (3 sets @ 15-20 reps)	141
		Crunch (3 sets @ 15-20 reps)	64
Tuesday	Off		
Wednesday	Total body	Dumbbell chest press (3 sets @ 15-20 reps)	53
		Dumbbell one-arm row (3 sets @ 15-20 reps)	35
		Dumbbell shoulder press (3 sets @ 15-20 reps)	81
		Dumbbell standing biceps curl (3 sets @ 15-20 reps)	92
		Cable triceps press-down (3 sets @ 15-20 reps)	110
		Barbell back squat (3 sets @ 15-20 reps)	121
		Lying leg curl (3 sets @ 15-20 reps)	136
		Machine standing calf raise (3 sets @ 15-20 reps)	141
		Crunch (3 sets @ 15-20 reps)	64
Thursday	Off		
Friday	Total body	Dumbbell chest press (3 sets @ 15-20 reps)	53
		Dumbbell one-arm row (3 sets @ 15-20 reps)	35
		Dumbbell shoulder press (3 sets @ 15-20 reps)	81
		Dumbbell standing biceps curl (3 sets @ 15-20 reps)	92
		Cable triceps press-down (3 sets @ 15-20 reps)	110
		Barbell back squat (3 sets @ 15-20 reps)	121
		Lying leg curl (3 sets @ 15-20 reps)	136
		Machine standing calf raise (3 sets @ 15-20 reps)	141
		Crunch (3 sets @ 15-20 reps)	64
Saturday	Off		
Sunday	Off		

Table 7.4   Break-In Week 3: Block 1 Microcycle 3

Perform these exercises at an RIR of 1 or 2.

DAY	TARGET MUSCLES	EXERCISES	PAGE
Monday	Total body	Dumbbell chest press (3 sets @ 15-20 reps)	53
		Dumbbell one-arm row (3 sets @ 15-20 reps)	35
		Dumbbell shoulder press (3 sets @ 15-20 reps)	81
		Dumbbell standing biceps curl (3 sets @ 15-20 reps)	92
		Cable triceps press-down (3 sets @ 15-20 reps)	110
		Barbell back squat (3 sets @ 15-20 reps)	121
		Lying leg curl (3 sets @ 15-20 reps)	136
		Machine standing calf raise (3 sets @ 15-20 reps)	141
		Crunch (3 sets @ 15-20 reps)	64
Tuesday	Off		
Wednesday	Total body	Dumbbell chest press (3 sets @ 15-20 reps)	53
		Dumbbell one-arm row (3 sets @ 15-20 reps)	35
		Dumbbell shoulder press (3 sets @ 15-20 reps)	81
		Dumbbell standing biceps curl (3 sets @ 15-20 reps)	92
		Cable triceps press-down (3 sets @ 15-20 reps)	110
		Barbell back squat (3 sets @ 15-20 reps)	121
		Lying leg curl (3 sets @ 15-20 reps)	136
		Machine standing calf raise (3 sets @ 15-20 reps)	141
		Crunch (3 sets @ 15-20 reps)	64
Thursday	Off		
Friday	Total body	Dumbbell chest press (3 sets @ 15-20 reps)	53
		Dumbbell one-arm row (3 sets @ 15-20 reps)	35
		Dumbbell shoulder press (3 sets @ 15-20 reps)	81
		Dumbbell standing biceps curl (3 sets @ 15-20 reps)	92
		Cable triceps press-down (3 sets @ 15-20 reps)	110
		Barbell back squat (3 sets @ 15-20 reps)	121
		Lying leg curl (3 sets @ 15-20 reps)	136
		Machine standing calf raise (3 sets @ 15-20 reps)	141
		Crunch (3 sets @ 15-20 reps)	64
Saturday	Off		
Sunday	Off		

Table 7.5   Break-In Week 4: Block 1 Microcycle 4

Perform these exercises at an RIR of approximately 4. Rest approximately two minutes between sets.

DAY	TARGET MUSCLES	EXERCISES	PAGE
Monday	Total body	Dumbbell chest press (3 sets @ 15-20 reps)	53
		Dumbbell one-arm row (3 sets @ 15-20 reps)	35
		Dumbbell shoulder press (3 sets @ 15-20 reps)	81
		Dumbbell standing biceps curl (3 sets @ 15-20 reps)	92
		Cable triceps press-down (3 sets @ 15-20 reps)	110
		Barbell back squat (3 sets @ 15-20 reps)	121
		Lying leg curl (3 sets @ 15-20 reps)	136
		Machine standing calf raise (3 sets @ 15-20 reps)	141
		Crunch (3 sets @ 15-20 reps)	64
Tuesday	Off		
Wednesday	Off		
Thursday	Total body	Dumbbell chest press (3 sets @ 15-20 reps)	53
		Dumbbell one-arm row (3 sets @ 15-20 reps)	35
		Dumbbell shoulder press (3 sets @ 15-20 reps)	81
		Dumbbell standing biceps curl (3 sets @ 15-20 reps)	92
		Cable triceps press-down (3 sets @ 15-20 reps)	110
		Barbell back squat (3 sets @ 15-20 reps)	121
		Lying leg curl (3 sets @ 15-20 reps)	136
		Machine standing calf raise (3 sets @ 15-20 reps)	141
		Crunch (3 sets @ 15-20 reps)	64
Friday	Off		
Saturday	Off		
Sunday	Off		

Table 7.6 Break-In Week 5: Block 2 Microcycle 1

Perform the first set of exercises at an RIR of about 3, perform the second set at an RIR of about 1 or 2, and take the final set to the point of concentric muscle failure. Rest 30 seconds between sets.

DAY	TARGET MUSCLES	EXERCISES	PAGE
Monday	Total body	Barbell chest press (3 sets @ 15-20 reps)	55
		Cable seated row (3 sets @ 15-20 reps)	41
		Military press (3 sets @ 15-20 reps)	80
		Barbell curl (3 sets @ 15-20 reps)	99
		Skull crusher (3 sets @ 15-20 reps)	106
		Bulgarian squat (3 sets @ 15-20 reps)	123
		Barbell stiff-legged deadlift (3 sets @ 15-20 reps)	129
		Machine standing calf raise (3 sets @ 15-20 reps)	141
		Cable rope kneeling crunch (3 sets @ 15-20 reps)	69
Tuesday	Off		
Wednesday	Total body	Dumbbell incline press (3 sets @ 15-20 reps)	51
		Lat pull-down (3 sets @ 15-20 reps)	46
		Dumbbell shoulder press (3 sets @ 15-20 reps)	81
		Dumbbell incline biceps curl (3 sets @ 15-20 reps)	93
		Cable rope overhead triceps extension (3 sets @ 15-20 reps)	105
		Barbell front squat (3 sets @ 15-20 reps)	120
		Machine seated leg curl (3 sets @ 15-20 reps)	138
		Machine seated calf raise (3 sets @ 15-20 reps)	140
		Bicycle crunch (3 sets @ 15-20 reps)	66
Thursday	Off		
Friday	Total body	Barbell incline press (3 sets @ 15-20 reps)	54
		Barbell overhand bent row (3 sets @ 15-20 reps)	38
		Cable upright row (3 sets @ 15-20 reps)	91
		Cable curl (3 sets @ 15-20 reps)	102
		Dumbbell overhead triceps extension (3 sets @ 15-20 reps)	104
		Dumbbell lunge (3 sets @ 15-20 reps)	116
		Good morning (3 sets @ 15-20 reps)	127
		Toe press (3 sets @ 15-20 reps)	139
		Reverse crunch (3 sets @ 15-20 reps)	65
Saturday	Off		
Sunday	Off		

Table 7.7   Break-In Week 6: Block 2 Microcycle 2

Perform the first set of exercises at an RIR of about 3, perform the second set at an RIR of about 1 or 2, and take the final set to the point of concentric muscle failure. Rest approximately two minutes between sets.

DAY	TARGET MUSCLES	EXERCISES	PAGE
Monday	Total body	Barbell chest press (3 sets @ 8-10 reps)	55
		Cable seated row (3 sets @ 8-10 reps)	41
		Military press (3 sets @ 8-10 reps)	80
		Barbell curl (3 sets @ 8-10 reps)	99
		Skull crusher (3 sets @ 8-10 reps)	106
		Bulgarian squat (3 sets @ 8-10 reps)	123
		Barbell stiff-legged deadlift (3 sets @ 8-10 reps)	129
		Machine standing calf raise (3 sets @ 8-10 reps)	141
		Cable rope kneeling crunch (3 sets @ 10-20 reps)	69
Tuesday	Off		
Wednesday	Total body	Dumbbell incline press (3 sets @ 8-10 reps)	51
		Lat pull-down (3 sets @ 8-10 reps)	46
		Dumbbell shoulder press (3 sets @ 8-10 reps)	81
		Dumbbell incline biceps curl (3 sets @ 8-10 reps)	93
		Cable rope overhead triceps extension (3 sets @ 8-10 reps)	105
		Barbell front squat (3 sets @ 8-10 reps)	120
		Machine seated leg curl (3 sets @ 8-10 reps)	138
		Machine seated calf raise (3 sets @ 8-10 reps)	140
		Bicycle crunch (3 sets @ 10-20 reps)	66
Thursday	Off		
Friday	Total body	Barbell incline press (3 sets @ 8-10 reps)	54
		Barbell overhand bent row (3 sets @ 8-10 reps)	38
		Cable upright row (3 sets @ 8-10 reps)	91
		Cable curl (3 sets @ 8-10 reps)	102
		Dumbbell overhead triceps extension (3 sets @ 8-10 reps)	104
		Dumbbell lunge (3 sets @ 8-10 reps)	116
		Good morning (3 sets @ 8-10 reps)	127
		Toe press (3 sets @ 8-10 reps)	139
		Reverse crunch (3 sets @ 10-20 reps)	65
Saturday	Off		
Sunday	Off		

Table 7.8   Break-In Week 7: Block 2 Microcycle 3

Perform the first set at an RIR of about 3, perform the second set at an RIR of about 2, and perform the final set at an RIR of about 1. Rest approximately three minutes between sets.

DAY	TARGET MUSCLES	EXERCISES	PAGE
Monday	Total body	Barbell chest press (3 sets @ 3-5 reps)	55
		Cable seated row (3 sets @ 3-5 reps)	41
		Military press (3 sets @ 3-5 reps)	80
		Barbell curl (3 sets @ 3-5 reps)	99
		Skull crusher (3 sets @ 3-5 reps)	106
		Bulgarian squat (3 sets @ 3-5 reps)	123
		Barbell stiff-legged deadlift (3 sets @ 3-5 reps)	129
		Machine standing calf raise (3 sets @ 3-5 reps)	141
		Cable rope kneeling crunch (3 sets @ 10-20 reps)	69
Tuesday	Off		
Wednesday	Total body	Dumbbell incline press (3 sets @ 3-5 reps)	51
		Lat pull-down (3 sets @ 3-5 reps)	46
		Dumbbell shoulder press (3 sets @ 3-5 reps)	81
		Dumbbell incline biceps curl (3 sets @ 3-5 reps)	93
		Cable rope overhead triceps extension (3 sets @ 3-5 reps)	105
		Barbell front squat (3 sets @ 3-5 reps)	120
		Machine seated leg curl (3 sets @ 3-5 reps)	138
		Machine seated calf raise (3 sets @ 3-5 reps)	140
		Bicycle crunch (3 sets @ 10-20 reps)	66
Thursday	Off		
Friday	Total body	Barbell incline press (3 sets @ 3-5 reps)	54
		Barbell overhand bent row (3 sets @ 3-5 reps)	38
		Cable upright row (3 sets @ 3-5 reps)	91
		Cable curl (3 sets @ 3-5 reps)	102
		Dumbbell overhead triceps extension (3 sets @ 3-5 reps)	104
		Dumbbell lunge (3 sets @ 3-5 reps)	116
		Good morning (3 sets @ 3-5 reps)	127
		Toe press (3 sets @ 3-5 reps)	139
		Reverse crunch (3 sets @ 10-20 reps)	65
Saturday	Off		
Sunday	Off		

Table 7.9   Break-In Week 8: Block 2 Microcycle 4

Perform these exercises at an RIR of approximately 4. Rest approximately two minutes between sets.

DAY	TARGET MUSCLES	EXERCISES	PAGE
Monday	Total body	Dumbbell chest press (3 sets @ 15-20 reps)	53
		Dumbbell one-arm row (3 sets @ 15-20 reps)	35
		Dumbbell shoulder press (3 sets @ 15-20 reps)	81
		Dumbbell standing biceps curl (3 sets @ 15-20 reps)	92
		Cable triceps press-down (3 sets @ 15-20 reps)	110
		Barbell back squat (3 sets @ 15-20 reps)	121
		Lying leg curl (3 sets @ 15-20 reps)	136
		Machine standing calf raise (3 sets @ 15-20 reps)	141
		Crunch (3 sets @ 15-20 reps)	64
Tuesday	Off		
Wednesday	Off		
Thursday	Total body	Barbell incline press (3 sets @ 15-20 reps)	54
		Barbell overhand bent row (3 sets @ 15-20 reps)	38
		Military press (3 sets @ 15-20 reps)	80
		Cable curl (3 sets @ 15-20 reps)	102
		Skull crusher (3 sets @ 15-20 reps)	106
		Barbell front squat (3 sets @ 15-20 reps)	120
		Barbell stiff-legged deadlift (3 sets @ 15-20 reps)	129
		Machine seated calf raise (3 sets @ 15-20 reps)	140
		Cable rope kneeling crunch (3 sets @ 15-20 reps)	69
Friday	Off		
Saturday	Off		
Sunday	Off		

CHAPTER 8

M.A.X. STRENGTH PHASE

The M.A.X. Muscle Plan begins with a strength phase. During this phase you'll focus on lifting heavy weights in a low rep range. The goal here is to get as strong as possible. It's a preparatory phase and thus hypertrophy is of secondary concern at this point, although you should generally gain some muscle depending on your training status.

Why is it important to build strength when the overall goal is to maximize muscle development? The short answer is that getting stronger ultimately fosters better muscle growth. I equate the process to building a house. Before erecting the frame of the house and laying down the hardwood flooring, you must first construct a rock-solid foundation. Without a strong foundation, the house will ultimately crumble. Similarly, to achieve maximal muscle development, you must build your body on a foundation of strength. Stronger muscles facilitate your ability to use heavier loads, and thus create greater mechanical tension, when performing moderate- to higher-rep sets. Given that mechanical tension is the primary mechanism driving hypertrophy, this in turn leads to greater muscular gains.

The most important adaptation to heavy lifting is an improvement in the response of your nervous system. You see, muscles are innervated—that is, activated—by nerve cells called neurons that transmit electrical and chemical signals to a given number of fibers within a muscle. A single neuron and all the corresponding fibers it innervates are called a motor unit. The major muscles in your body are innervated by multiple motor units, often many thousands.

How does all this physiology relate to muscle growth? The ability of your muscles to exert force is governed by three distinct neural mechanisms: recruitment, rate coding, and synchronization. Let's take a brief look at how heavy strength training affects each of these factors.

Recruitment refers to the ability of your nervous system to activate motor units. Recruitment is generally governed by the size principle, which suggests that smaller motor units (primarily made up of endurance-oriented slow-twitch fibers) are recruited first and that larger motor units (primarily made up of strength-oriented fast-twitch fibers) are progressively recruited thereafter if and when additional force is required. Although studies show that full motor unit recruitment occurs in most large muscles at approximately 80-90 percent of maximal voluntary contraction (2, 4), some believe that very heavy weight training may help condition stubborn high-threshold motor units, thereby allowing their recruitment at lower percentages of 1RM. Hypothetically, this leads to greater muscle fatigue across the full spectrum of fibers and thus greater muscle growth.

Rate coding refers to the frequency at which nerve impulses are stimulated during a lift. Nerve impulses that fire with a high frequency produce more muscle tension than do lower-frequency impulses. Rate coding is widely considered the most important determinant of your ability to produce force. The good news is that heavy strength training increases the rate at which nerve impulses fire, and it can extend the firing period. The upshot is a greater sustained mechanical tension during your lifts.

Synchronization refers to the coordinated timing between different motor units within a muscle (intramuscular coordination) or between different synergists (intermuscular coordination). As an analogy, think of synchronization as similar to a symphony orchestra. If the string section is not in sync with the percussion section (analogous to intermuscular coordination) or the violins are not in sync with each other (analogous to intramuscular coordination), the end result is a hodgepodge of sounds. To produce sweet music, all the instruments must play harmoniously. Similarly, if the impulses reaching different motor units are out of sync, then muscle force is compromised. Fibers must contract as a unit in precise accord to maximize force production. Heavy lifting helps foster both intramuscular and intermuscular harmony between fibers, both in the target muscles and the stabilizing muscles.

By enhancing the efficiency of recruitment, rate coding, and synchronization, the M.A.X. strength phase lays the groundwork for future muscle growth. It provides a strong base on which to build your body. As long as you follow the guidelines laid out herein in a step-by-step fashion, you'll set the stage for maximizing your muscular potential.

PROGRAM PROTOCOL

The M.A.X. strength phase is an eight-week, heavy-load mesocycle that consists of two training blocks. Each block includes four one-week microcycles. Block 1 uses a total-body routine that works all the major muscles during each session, and block 2 uses a split routine that divides training into upper-body and lower-body sessions (except week 8, which is a total-body deload). Blocks are structured to progressively increase training volume over the course of the mesocycle while maintaining intensity of load.

With the exception of assistance exercises, you'll train in a range of one to five reps and rest three to five minutes between sets. Three sets are performed per exercise. The goal is to optimize force production by lifting heavy and hard. Realize, though, that constantly grinding out reps at near-maximal intensities really takes a toll on the body. Over time, it can overtax your neuromuscular system and overstress your joints. To counteract these potential negative effects, the load and volume are carefully manipulated throughout the training cycle, with deload periods interspersed at regimented points to allow adequate recuperation and promote restoration. What's more, sets are mostly terminated before reaching failure; all-out training is not needed to optimize strength gains and potentially can be counterproductive (1). That said, I have suggested you may potentially choose to make a maximal attempt on the 1RM sets as a means to assess strength progress. Note, however, failure training is not mandatory in this phase. Discretion should be employed when attempting to train to failure with very heavy loads, balancing the individual risks with the potential rewards.

Lifts can be categorized as either primary exercises or accessory exercises. Primary exercises are multi-joint movements that tax the prime movers and require a significant contribution from the muscles that assist the prime movers (synergists) and the muscles that stabilize the body during the performance of the exercise (stabilizers). In other words, they involve large amounts of total-body muscle mass. Examples include variations of squats, rows, and presses. These movements lend themselves to maximal or near-maximal lifts and thus are most conducive to optimizing increases in absolute strength.

Accessory exercises, on the other hand, generally refer to single-joint movements that involve working smaller amounts of muscle mass. In the context of the M.A.X. strength phase, accessory exercises help to rectify muscle imbalances by preventing weak links from forming in the kinetic chain. By their nature, primary exercises tend to stress certain muscles more than others. In the squat, for example, hamstring activity is only about 50 percent that of the quadriceps (3). If you don't perform direct hamstring work, chances are you'll become quad dominant and impair muscle symmetry. Thus, consider accessory exercises to be complementary movements that fill in the "muscular gaps" left by primary exercises.

One caveat: Because accessory exercises place greater stress on joints, they tend to be incompatible with the use of very heavy loads. Hence, it's preferable to use a slightly higher rep range (approximately six to eight reps per set) for these movements when training for strength.

Exercise selection is rather limited in the M.A.X. strength phase. Although exercise variety is important for maximizing muscle hypertrophy, it is less relevant with respect to strength development. The reason? Consistently training the same lifts hardwires neuromuscular patterns, thus enhancing both intra- and intermuscular coordination. Because strength gains are highly dependent on neuromuscular efficiency, strength is best maximized by performing the same basic movements on a regular basis.

You should regulate tempo on both the concentric and eccentric portions of each rep. Concentrically, your objective is to lift as explosively as possible. Given that loads approach repetition maximum (i.e., the maximum amount you can lift once but not twice with proper form), this is easier said than done. You can put all your effort into producing force, but the weights won't move very fast. This isn't of concern; as long as your *intent* is to lift explosively, you'll derive the desired strength-related benefits. On the other hand, perform eccentric repetitions a bit more slowly. Aim for a cadence of approximately two to three seconds. The most important consideration is to stay controlled so that you do not compromise form. Never bounce at the bottom of a movement; you might eke out an extra rep or two, but you'll overstress your joints in a way that's bound to lead to injury.

It is important, but contrary to hypertrophy-oriented training, to employ an external attentional focus during the concentric portion of lifts. Simply stated, an external focus involves visualizing the outcome of the movement; in this case, completing the lift. As previously mentioned, an external focus reigns supreme when it comes to strength- and power-related tasks. Accordingly, set your mind to think externally throughout this phase. Cues such as "push your feet through the floor" when performing a squat or "drive the bar through the ceiling" when performing a shoulder press are examples of how you can optimize focus during strength-oriented lifts.

You'll notice that the arms are not trained directly in the strength phase, and ab work is substantially curtailed. Before some of you cry heresy, hear out my rationale. Remember that the goal of this phase is to get strong. Because you have limited recuperative abilities, all your resources should be centered on the large muscle group lifts that contribute most to increases in strength. The arms and abs don't fall into this category, and training them directly would only take away valuable energy better reserved for maximal strength development. Remember, you have limited resources for coping with the stress of intense exercise; use them wisely.

In case you're worried that these muscles will somehow shrivel up if you don't work them directly, rest easy. The biceps and triceps are heavily involved in all the structural lifts as well as many of the assistance lifts, and the muscles of the core act as stabilizers in virtually every exercise you perform. Hence, they receive ample work throughout the strength mesocycle—more than enough to maintain or even improve development. I've carried out numerous studies in resistance-trained individuals who've achieved significant increases in arm development performing just multi-joint upper-body exercises (5, 6). And rest assured that you will blitz these muscle groups during the later phases of the program to achieve the coveted cannonball biceps and six-pack abs.

PROGRAM SPECIFICS

As noted, the M.A.X. strength phase is an eight-week mesocycle that comprises two training blocks. Each block uses a technique called step loading in which the magnitude of load progressively increases over each of the first three weeks; during this period, you should attempt to increase the amount of weight used at the prescribed rep range without compromising form. The fourth week consists of a deload microcycle of low-intensity, low-volume training. The deload periods allow you to restore and rejuvenate muscles, joints, and ultimately your body as a whole, helping to facilitate recovery and stave off the potential for overtraining. Here are the particulars of each block.

BLOCK 1

Block 1 is composed of four one-week microcycles. During the first three microcycles, you'll work out on three nonconsecutive days per week (e.g., Monday, Wednesday, and Friday) and follow a total-body routine that trains all the major muscle groups during each session. One exercise will be performed per muscle group. You'll perform three sets per exercise and rest approximately three to five minutes between sets. The following step-loading progression will be employed.

The first microcycle in block 1 (week 1 of the mesocycle) employs a loading range of four to five reps. Your level of effort on all sets should correspond to an RIR of 2 or 3, meaning that the lifts are fairly taxing.

The second microcycle in block 1 (week 2) employs a loading range of two to three reps. Your level of effort on all sets should correspond to an RIR of 1 or 2, meaning that the lifts are highly taxing but do not progress to all-out muscle failure.

The third microcycle in block 1 (week 3) employs a loading range of one to five reps in a descending-set fashion. In the first set you'll perform four to five reps, in the second set you'll perform two to three, and the final set targets a near-maximal lift at approximately 1RM. Perform the first set at an RIR of 2, the second set at an RIR of 1, and the final set can be taken to the point of concentric muscle failure, or, if desired, you can leave one-half rep or so in the tank (i.e., where you could have ground out another rep with less than ideal form).

The fourth microcycle in block 1 (week 4) is a deload. You'll train two days per week, allowing 72 hours between sessions (e.g., Monday and Thursday or Tuesday and Friday), and follow a total-body routine that works all the major muscle groups during each session. You'll perform one exercise of three sets per muscle group at a loading zone of 15-20 reps. Sets should not be overly challenging; aim for an RIR of 4 or so. If you're struggling on the last rep, lighten the weight!

BLOCK 2

Block 2 is composed of four one-week microcycles. During the first three microcycles, you'll train four days per week using a sequence of either two on, one off, two on, two off (e.g., Monday, Tuesday, Thursday, and Friday) or two on, one off, one on, one off, one on, one off (e.g., Monday, Tuesday, Thursday, and Saturday). The block incorporates a two-day split where you work the upper body on days 1 and 3, and the lower body on days 2 and 4. The number of exercises per muscle group increases to include both a primary lift and a corresponding assistance exercise. You'll perform three sets per exercise and rest approximately three to five minutes between sets on the primary exercises and two minutes on the assistance exercises. Loading is carried out using the same step-loading progression as in block 1. Thus, volume increases while rep ranges remain constant.

The first microcycle in block 2 (week 5 of the mesocycle) employs a loading range of four to five reps for the primary exercises and six to eight reps for the assistance exercises. Your level of effort on all sets should correspond to an RIR of 2 or 3, meaning that the lifts are taxing but not overly stressful.

The second microcycle in block 2 (week 6) employs a loading range of two to three reps for the primary exercises and six to eight reps for the assistance exercises. Your level of effort on all sets should correspond to an RIR of 1 or 2, meaning that the lifts are very taxing but do not progress to the point of muscle failure.

The third microcycle in block 2 (week 7) employs a loading range of one to five reps in a descending-set fashion for the primary exercises. Thus, the first set for each primary exercise targets four to five reps, the second set targets two to three reps, and the final set targets a single lift. On these sets, perform the first set at an RIR of 2, the second set at an RIR of 1, and on the final set, either train to the point of concentric muscle failure or leave one-half rep or so in the tank (i.e., where you could have ground out another rep with less than ideal form). Assistance exercises will maintain a six to eight rep range for all sets, and effort should correspond to an RIR of approximately 1 or 2; do not go to failure on the assistance exercises.

The fourth microcycle in block 2 (week 8) is a deload. You'll train two days per week, allowing 72 hours between sessions (e.g., Monday and Thursday), and follow a total-body routine that works all the major muscle groups during each session. You'll perform one exercise of three sets per muscle group at a loading range of 15-20 reps. Sets should not be overly challenging; aim for an RIR of 4 or so. If you're struggling on the last few reps, lighten the weight!

Table 8.1 summarizes the strength phase protocol, and sample routines (tables 8.2 through 8.9) are provided on the subsequent pages. These routines should serve as a basic template for constructing your workouts. Modify specific exercises according to your individual needs and abilities.

Table 8.1   Summary of Strength Protocol

TRAINING VARIABLE	PROTOCOL
Repetitions	Structural exercises: 1-5
	Assistance exercises: 6-8
Sets	3 per exercise
Rest interval	Structural exercises: 3-5 min
	Assistance exercises: 2 min
Tempo	Concentric: explosive intent
	Eccentric: 2-3 sec
Frequency	3-4 days per week

Table 8.2 Strength Phase Week 1: Block 1 Microcycle 1

Perform these exercises at an RIR of 2 or 3.

DAY	TARGET MUSCLES	EXERCISES	PAGE
Monday	Total body	Military press (3 sets @ 4-5 reps)	80
		Barbell reverse-grip bent row (3 sets @ 4-5 reps)	37
		Barbell chest press (3 sets @ 4-5 reps)	55
		Deadlift (3 sets @ 4-5 reps)	125
		Barbell back squat (3 sets @ 4-5 reps)	121
Tuesday	Off		
Wednesday	Total body	Military press (3 sets @ 4-5 reps)	80
		Barbell reverse-grip bent row (3 sets @ 4-5 reps)	37
		Barbell chest press (3 sets @ 4-5 reps)	55
		Deadlift (3 sets @ 4-5 reps)	125
		Barbell back squat (3 sets @ 4-5 reps)	121
Thursday	Off		
Friday	Total body	Military press (3 sets @ 4-5 reps)	80
		Barbell reverse-grip bent row (3 sets @ 4-5 reps)	37
		Barbell chest press (3 sets @ 4-5 reps)	55
		Deadlift (3 sets @ 4-5 reps)	125
		Barbell back squat (3 sets @ 4-5 reps)	121
Saturday	Off		
Sunday	Off		

Table 8.3   Strength Phase Week 2: Block 1 Microcycle 2

Perform these exercises at an RIR of 1 or 2.

DAY	TARGET MUSCLES	EXERCISES	PAGE
Monday	Total body	Military press (3 sets @ 2-3 reps)	80
		Barbell reverse-grip bent row (3 sets @ 2-3 reps)	37
		Barbell chest press (3 sets @ 2-3 reps)	55
		Deadlift (3 sets @ 2-3 reps)	125
		Barbell back squat (3 sets @ 2-3 reps)	121
Tuesday	Off		
Wednesday	Total body	Military press (3 sets @ 2-3 reps)	80
		Barbell reverse-grip bent row (3 sets @ 2-3 reps)	37
		Barbell chest press (3 sets @ 2-3 reps)	55
		Deadlift (3 sets @ 2-3 reps)	125
		Barbell back squat (3 sets @ 2-3 reps)	121
Thursday	Off		
Friday	Total body	Military press (3 sets @ 2-3 reps)	80
		Barbell reverse-grip bent row (3 sets @ 2-3 reps)	37
		Barbell chest press (3 sets @ 2-3 reps)	55
		Deadlift (3 sets @ 2-3 reps)	125
		Barbell back squat (3 sets @ 2-3 reps)	121
Saturday	Off		
Sunday	Off		

Table 8.4 Strength Phase Week 3: Block 1 Microcycle 3

Perform the first set of exercises at an RIR of 2, perform the second set at an RIR of 1, and take the final maximal set to the point of concentric muscle failure or just short of failure (RIR of 0.5).

DAY	TARGET MUSCLES	EXERCISES	PAGE
Monday	Total body	Military press (3 sets @ 4-5 reps, 2-3 reps, 1 rep)	80
		Barbell reverse-grip bent row (3 sets @ 4-5 reps, 2-3 reps, 1 rep)	37
		Barbell chest press (3 sets @ 4-5 reps, 2-3 reps, 1 rep)	55
		Deadlift (3 sets @ 4-5 reps, 2-3 reps, 1 rep)	125
		Barbell back squat (3 sets @ 4-5 reps, 2-3 reps, 1 rep)	121
Tuesday	Off		
Wednesday	Total body	Military press (3 sets @ 4-5 reps, 2-3 reps, 1 rep)	80
		Barbell reverse-grip bent row (3 sets @ 4-5 reps, 2-3 reps, 1 rep)	37
		Barbell chest press (3 sets @ 4-5 reps, 2-3 reps, 1 rep)	55
		Deadlift (3 sets @ 4-5 reps, 2-3 reps, 1 rep)	125
		Barbell back squat (3 sets @ 4-5 reps, 2-3 reps, 1 rep)	121
Thursday	Off		
Friday	Total body	Military press (3 sets @ 4-5 reps, 2-3 reps, 1 rep)	80
		Barbell reverse-grip bent row (3 sets @ 4-5 reps, 2-3 reps, 1 rep)	37
		Barbell chest press (3 sets @ 4-5 reps, 2-3 reps, 1 rep)	55
		Deadlift (3 sets @ 4-5 reps, 2-3 reps, 1 rep)	125
		Barbell back squat (3 sets @ 4-5 reps, 2-3 reps, 1 rep)	121
Saturday	Off		
Sunday	Off		

Table 8.5   Strength Phase Week 4: Block 1 Microcycle 4

Perform these exercises at an RIR of about 4.

DAY	TARGET MUSCLES	EXERCISES	PAGE
Monday	Total body	Dumbbell incline fly (3 sets @ 15-20 reps)	60
		Lat pull-down (3 sets @ 15-20 reps)	46
		Barbell upright row (3 sets @ 15-20 reps)	90
		Bulgarian squat (3 sets @ 15-20 reps)	123
		Lying leg curl (3 sets @ 15-20 reps)	136
		Machine standing calf raise (3 sets @ 15-20 reps)	141
		Plank (3 sets @ 30 sec static hold)	72
Tuesday	Off		
Wednesday	Off		
Thursday	Total body	Cable fly (3 sets @ 15-20 reps)	62
		Cable seated row (3 sets @ 15-20 reps)	41
		Dumbbell lateral raise (3 sets @ 15-20 reps)	83
		Dumbbell reverse lunge (3 sets @ 15-20 reps)	117
		Machine seated leg curl (3 sets @ 15-20 reps)	138
		Toe press (3 sets @ 15-20 reps)	139
		Side bridge (3 sets @ 30 sec static hold)	73
Friday	Off		
Saturday	Off		
Sunday	Off		

Table 8.6   Strength Phase Week 5: Block 2 Microcycle 1

Perform these exercises at an RIR of 2 or 3.

DAY	TARGET MUSCLES	EXERCISES	PAGE
Monday	Upper body	Military press (3 sets @ 4-5 reps)	80
		Dumbbell lateral raise (3 sets @ 6-8 reps)	83
		Barbell reverse-grip bent row (3 sets @ 4-5 reps)	37
		Lat pull-down (3 sets @ 6-8 reps)	46
		Barbell chest press (3 sets @ 4-5 reps)	55
		Dumbbell incline fly (3 sets @ 6-8 reps)	60
Tuesday	Lower body	Deadlift (3 sets @ 4-5 reps)	125
		Barbell back squat (3 sets @ 4-5 reps)	121
		Good morning (3 sets @ 6-8 reps)	127
		Lying leg curl (3 sets @ 6-8 reps)	136
		Machine standing calf raise (3 sets @ 6-8 reps)	141
Wednesday	Off		
Thursday	Upper body	Military press (3 sets @ 4-5 reps)	80
		Cable lateral raise (3 sets @ 6-8 reps)	85
		Barbell reverse-grip bent row (3 sets @ 4-5 reps)	37
		Chin-up (3 sets @ 6-8 reps)	44
		Barbell chest press (3 sets @ 4-5 reps)	55
		Cable fly (3 sets @ 6-8 reps)	62
Friday	Lower body	Deadlift (3 sets @ 4-5 reps)	125
		Barbell back squat (3 sets @ 4-5 reps)	121
		Barbell stiff-legged deadlift (3 sets @ 6-8 reps)	129
		Machine seated leg curl (3 sets @ 6-8 reps)	138
		Toe press (3 sets @ 6-8 reps)	139
Saturday	Off		
Sunday	Off		

Table 8.7   Strength Phase Week 6: Block 2 Microcycle 2

Perform these exercises at an RIR of 1 or 2.

DAY	TARGET MUSCLES	EXERCISES	PAGE
Monday	Upper body	Military press (3 sets @ 2-3 reps)	80
		Dumbbell lateral raise (3 sets @ 6-8 reps)	83
		Barbell reverse-grip bent row (3 sets @ 2-3 reps)	37
		Lat pull-down (3 sets @ 6-8 reps)	46
		Barbell chest press (3 sets @ 2-3 reps)	55
		Dumbbell incline fly (3 sets @ 6-8 reps)	60
Tuesday	Lower body	Deadlift (3 sets @ 2-3 reps)	125
		Barbell back squat (3 sets @ 2-3 reps)	121
		Good morning (3 sets @ 6-8 reps)	127
		Lying leg curl (3 sets @ 6-8 reps)	136
		Machine standing calf raise (3 sets @ 6-8 reps)	141
Wednesday	Off		
Thursday	Upper body	Military press (3 sets @ 2-3 reps)	80
		Cable lateral raise (3 sets @ 6-8 reps)	85
		Barbell reverse-grip bent row (3 sets @ 2-3 reps)	37
		Chin-up (3 sets @ 6-8 reps)	44
		Barbell chest press (3 sets @ 2-3 reps)	55
		Cable fly (3 sets @ 6-8 reps)	62
Friday	Lower body	Deadlift (3 sets @ 2-3 reps)	125
		Barbell back squat (3 sets @ 2-3 reps)	121
		Barbell stiff-legged deadlift (3 sets @ 6-8 reps)	129
		Machine seated leg curl (3 sets @ 6-8 reps)	138
		Toe press (3 sets @ 6-8 reps)	139
Saturday	Off		
Sunday	Off		

Table 8.8 Strength Phase Week 7: Block 2 Microcycle 3

On the primary exercises, the first set should be performed at an RIR of 2, the second set should be performed at an RIR of 1, and the final set should be taken to the point of concentric muscle failure or just short of failure (RIR of 0.5). Assistance exercises should be performed at an RIR of approximately 1 or 2.

DAY	TARGET MUSCLES	EXERCISES	PAGE
Monday	Upper body	Military press (3 sets @ 4-5 reps, 2-3 reps, 1 rep)	80
		Dumbbell lateral raise (3 sets @ 6-8 reps)	83
		Barbell reverse-grip bent row (3 sets @ 4-5 reps, 2-3 reps, 1 rep)	37
		Lat pull-down (3 sets @ 6-8 reps)	46
		Barbell chest press (3 sets @ 4-5 reps, 2-3 reps, 1 rep)	55
		Dumbbell incline fly (3 sets @ 6-8 reps)	60
Tuesday	Lower body	Deadlift (3 sets @ 4-5 reps, 2-3 reps, 1 rep)	125
		Barbell back squat (3 sets @ 4-5 reps, 2-3 reps, 1 rep)	121
		Good morning (3 sets @ 6-8 reps)	127
		Lying leg curl (3 sets @ 6-8 reps)	136
		Machine standing calf raise (3 sets @ 6-8 reps)	141
Wednesday	Off		
Thursday	Upper body	Military press (3 sets @ 4-5 reps, 2-3 reps, 1 rep)	80
		Cable lateral raise (3 sets @ 6-8 reps)	85
		Barbell reverse-grip bent row (3 sets @ 4-5 reps, 2-3 reps, 1 rep)	37
		Chin-up (3 sets @ 6-8 reps)	44
		Barbell chest press (3 sets @ 4-5 reps, 2-3 reps, 1 rep)	55
		Cable fly (3 sets @ 6-8 reps)	62
Friday	Lower body	Deadlift (3 sets @ 4-5 reps, 2-3 reps, 1 rep)	125
		Barbell back squat (3 sets @ 4-5 reps, 2-3 reps, 1 rep)	121
		Barbell stiff-legged deadlift (3 sets @ 6-8 reps)	129
		Machine seated leg curl (3 sets @ 6-8 reps)	138
		Toe press (3 sets @ 6-8 reps)	139
Saturday	Off		
Sunday	Off		

Table 8.9   Strength Phase Week 8: Block 2 Microcycle 4

Perform these exercises at an RIR of about 4.

DAY	TARGET MUSCLES	EXERCISES	PAGE
Monday	Total body	Dumbbell incline fly (3 sets @ 15-20 reps)	60
		Lat pull-down (3 sets @ 15-20 reps)	46
		Barbell upright row (3 sets @ 15-20 reps)	90
		Bulgarian squat (3 sets @ 15-20 reps)	123
		Lying leg curl (3 sets @ 15-20 reps)	136
		Machine standing calf raise (3 sets @ 15-20 reps)	141
		Plank (3 sets @ 30 sec static hold)	72
Tuesday	Off		
Wednesday	Off		
Thursday	Total body	Cable fly (3 sets @ 15-20 reps)	62
		Cable seated row (3 sets @ 15-20 reps)	41
		Dumbbell lateral raise (3 sets @ 15-20 reps)	83
		Dumbbell reverse lunge (3 sets @ 15-20 reps)	117
		Machine seated leg curl (3 sets @ 15-20 reps)	138
		Toe press (3 sets @ 15-20 reps)	139
		Side bridge (3 sets @ 30 sec static hold)	73
Friday	Off		
Saturday	Off		
Sunday	Off		

M.A.X.
METABOLIC PHASE

The metabolic phase is a preparatory phase that conditions your body for hypertrophy training. The goal here is to optimize training efficiency by packing more exercise into less time, i.e., increasing training density. This is accomplished by training with a combination of high repetitions (15-30 reps per set) and short rest intervals (approximately 30 seconds or less). Rest intervals progressively decrease over the course of the cycle to bring about the desired metabolic adaptations.

Although the hypertrophic benefits of metabolic training may not be readily apparent, it indeed can have positive effects on muscle development. First and foremost, metabolic training increases your lactate threshold, the point at which lactic acid begins to rapidly accumulate in working muscles. From a muscle-building standpoint, lactic acid is a double-edged sword. On one hand, there is evidence that it serves to stimulate hypertrophy, at least in animal models (5-7). Although the mechanisms are not entirely clear, lactate conceivably may function as a signaling agent that turns on intracellular anabolic pathways. On the other hand, excessive buildup of lactic acid (specifically the hydrogen ions) can interfere with muscle contraction, thus reducing the number of reps you can perform in a set. Here's where metabolic training comes into play. Adaptations associated with metabolic training include an increase in the number of capillaries (tiny blood vessels that facilitate the exchange of nutrients and metabolic waste) and an improved muscle-buffering capacity, both of which help delay lactic buildup. The upshot is that you're able to maintain greater time under tension at a given workload without compromising the proposed hypertrophy-related benefits of lactate accumulation. In addition, you develop a greater tolerance for higher volumes of work—an important component of maximizing hypertrophy.

Metabolic training also improves glycogen storage capacity. Glycogen is the term for stored carbohydrate. The majority of glycogen is stored in muscle tissue, with the balance deposited in liver cells. Here's the kicker: Each gram of stored glycogen attracts 3 grams of water into the muscle. Increase muscle glycogen stores and you increase overall muscle size, a phenomenon called sarcoplasmic hypertrophy. Although sarcoplasmic hypertrophy does not meaningfully contribute to strength capacity, it does enhance muscular aesthetics, improving the overall shape of your physique. If you aspire to maximize muscular gains, sarcoplasmic hypertrophy is your ally.

In addition, metabolic training boosts your recovery ability. As mentioned, training in a metabolic fashion increases the network of capillaries that deliver nutrients and other substances (such as oxygen, hormones, and so on) to body tissues. A greater capillary density allows for greater nutrient transfer to your muscles. This facilitates better recovery after an intense workout in that it supplies damaged muscles with the necessary materials for remodeling.

Finally, metabolic training may help to fully stimulate the growth of slow-twitch (i.e., type I) muscle fibers (4). Research remains inconclusive on the topic, but there is some evidence that these fibers might respond better to higher rep ranges given their endurance-oriented nature. Although slow-twitch fibers are often dismissed as inconsequential from a muscle-building standpoint, don't discount their importance to overall muscle development. Superior slow-twitch fiber hypertrophy is one of the hypothesized reasons bodybuilders display greater muscularity compared with powerlifters (3). To maximize muscle size, it is necessary to maximally stimulate the full spectrum of fibers, including slow-twitch fibers.

Before you conclude that including extended cycles of metabolic conditioning in a hypertrophy program is beneficial, remember that this type of training is intended to set the stage for muscle development, not to maximize hypertrophy. In fact, metabolic training potentially can negatively affect strength gains made in the previous phase if carried out over a prolonged time frame. Thus, limit metabolic cycles to relatively short time periods (i.e., four weeks) to avoid any detrimental impact on force-producing capacity.

Moreover, the weights used in this phase are comparatively light, but that doesn't mean the workouts will be a walk in the park. Quite the contrary. Metabolic training can be even more physically and mentally demanding than heavy weight training. Pushing past the intense burn that continues to build up during a high-rep set requires a high tolerance for discomfort and lots of resolve. It's definitely not for the weak of mind!

PROGRAM PROTOCOL

The metabolic phase of the M.A.X. Muscle Plan is a four-week, low-load mesocycle consisting of a single training block. It's long enough to promote desired metabolic adaptations without compromising muscle strength. Three metabolic training strategies are employed on successive weeks, sequentially arranged to heighten metabolic accumulation over the course of the mesocycle. Here is an overview of each strategy.

1. **Straight-set metabolic training.** Straight-set metabolic training is similar to traditional strength training: You perform a given number of sets for an exercise, proceed to the next exercise for a given number

of sets (for our purposes herein, you perform three sets), and so on until you've completed the routine. Simple, right? The unique aspect of straight-set metabolic training is that repetitions are maintained in the high range (15-30 reps per set) and rest intervals are very brief (30 seconds between sets). This results in high amounts of metabolic stress that cause an intense burning sensation in the working muscles. Because rest periods are short, your body won't have sufficient time to fully recover. Thus, you'll need to progressively decrease the amount of weight used in the second and third sets of an exercise to maintain the target rep range. Don't be concerned. Remember, the goal of metabolic training is to increase your lactate threshold and promote slow-twitch fiber hypertrophy; the load is of secondary consequence.

2. **Paired-set training.** A superset is defined as two exercises performed in succession without rest. From a metabolic-conditioning standpoint, one of the best superset methods is paired-set training. This technique supersets exercises that share an agonist–antagonist relationship, meaning that when one muscle contracts, the muscle on the opposing side of the body relaxes. Evidence shows the strategy hastens the onset of metabolic fatigue, particularly when employing relatively short rest intervals (1). Although paired-set training often focuses on opposing muscle groups (e.g., back and chest, biceps and triceps, quads and hamstrings), you'll base exercising pairings on opposing joint actions such as flexion–extension and abduction–adduction. Plantarflexion (e.g., calf raises) and spinal flexion (e.g., crunches) are not paired because their antagonist movements (dorsiflexion and spinal hyperextension, respectively) are of limited utility to hypertrophy-oriented routines.

To ensure optimal efficiency, set up exercise stations in advance so that you are able to move quickly between exercises. You'll perform a set of the first exercise, proceed directly to the second movement as quickly as possible, rest for approximately 30 seconds, and then repeat for two additional supersets. Once you complete a given superset, move on to the next agonist–antagonist pairing and so on until you complete all paired sets.

3. **Circuit training.** As opposed to straight-set training, circuit training requires that you move from one exercise to the next with minimal rest (ideally less than 10 seconds). In essence, you perform one giant set of multiple exercises for different muscle groups. To facilitate your ability to transition swiftly between movements, set up in advance a series of exercise stations that work muscles in a push–pull fashion. Start with upper-body exercises and proceed to movements for the lower body; perform abdominal exercises last in the sequence (i.e., chest, back, shoulders, biceps, triceps, quads, hamstrings, calves, abdomen). After finishing the circuit, go back to the first exercise and perform two additional circuits in the same expeditious fashion. Rest approximately one to two minutes between circuits.

You'll perform three sets per muscle group and follow a total-body routine that works all the major muscles during each session. The key to optimizing results is to train at high levels of effort; you don't need to take sets to the point of muscle failure, but they must be very challenging. It's important to "feel the burn" as you reach the last few reps of a set. This burning sensation indicates that you're accumulating metabolites (i.e., lactic acid). If you aren't sufficiently pushing yourself to complete each set, the metabolic effect will be compromised.

Multi-joint exercises are incorporated into the routine whenever possible. Research shows that the metabolic cost of an exercise is directly related to the amount of muscle worked (2). In other words, involve more muscle and you increase metabolic stress. Thus, squats, rows, presses, and the like are used to work the muscles of the torso and thighs; single-joint movements are reserved for the muscles of the arms and calves.

Machine-based exercises are particularly well-suited for this phase because their use reduces instability and thus can help avoid the breakdown in form that inevitably accompanies heightened metabolic acidosis. However, lining up the necessary machines in a gym for efficient performance can be logistically infeasible; moreover, those training at home often don't have access to such equipment. If so, it's fine to substitute comparable free weight exercises; just be extra careful with your form as you approach the end of the set. It's never a good trade-off to compromise technique in an effort to grind out an extra rep or two, particularly when you're metabolically fatigued.

To condition as many muscle fibers as possible, you'll perform a greater variety of exercises during this phase than during the strength phase. Considering that you will perform sets with limited rest, this can be a challenge if you work out in a crowded gym. In this case, simply substitute a comparable exercise that targets similar muscles. Minimizing rest intervals is far and away the most important objective. If you have to sacrifice some variety to achieve greater expediency, so be it.

Perform repetitions using a mind–muscle connection throughout the concentric and eccentric portions of each rep. This not only will help to optimize metabolic conditioning but also hones your ability to focus on the target muscles during training. This skill will serve you well when progressing to the muscle phase of the program.

PROGRAM SPECIFICS

The metabolic phase consists of a single training block made up of four one-week microcycles. Rest intervals between sets progressively decrease over the first three microcycles to generate increased metabolic stress; volume stays relatively constant. A step-loading approach is employed whereby loads get progressively lighter over the course of each microcycle. The final week is a low-volume deload microcycle intended to restore and rejuvenate your body. Here are the particulars for each microcycle.

The first microcycle (week 1 of the mesocycle) incorporates straight-set metabolic training. Carry out the first set at an RIR of 3, the second at an RIR of 2, and the final set at an RIR of 1. Aim for 15-30 reps per set. If you can't perform the minimum number of reps, lighten the weight; if you can perform more than the maximum number of reps, increase the weight. Rest about 30 seconds between sets—just long enough to catch your breath. After finishing all three sets of an exercise, move quickly to the next exercise, taking no more than about 30 seconds between movements.

The second microcycle (week 2) incorporates reciprocal supersets. Carry out the first set at an RIR of 3, the second at an RIR of 2, and the final set at an RIR of 1. Aim for 15-30 reps per set. If you can't perform the minimum number of reps, lighten the weight; if you can perform more than the maximum number of reps, increase the weight. Take approximately 30 seconds of rest between each superset. After finishing all three sets of a superset combo, move quickly to the next superset, taking no more than 30 seconds between movements.

The third microcycle (week 3) incorporates circuit training. Carry out the first set at an RIR of 3, the second at an RIR of 2, and the final set at an RIR of 1. Aim for 15-30 reps per set. If you can't perform the minimum number of reps, lighten the weight; if you can perform more than the maximum number of reps, increase the weight. Move from one exercise to the next as quickly as possible; keep rest to an absolute minimum—ideally ten seconds or less. After finishing the entire circuit, rest approximately one to two minutes, then repeat the process two more times, again resting as little as possible during each circuit.

The fourth microcycle (week 4) is a deload. You'll train two days per week, allowing 72 hours between sessions (e.g., Monday and Thursday), and follow a total-body routine that works all the major muscle groups during each session. One exercise of three sets will be performed per muscle group, with loads equating to 15-20 reps. Effort should equate to an RIR of about 4.

Table 9.1 summarizes the metabolic phase protocol, and sample routines (tables 9.2 through 9.5) are provided on the subsequent pages. These routines should serve as a basic template for constructing your workouts. Modify specific exercises according to your individual needs and abilities.

Table 9.1   Summary of Metabolic Protocol

TRAINING VARIABLE	PROTOCOL
Repetitions	15-30
Sets	3 per exercise
Rest interval	30 sec or less
Tempo	Mind–muscle connection
Frequency	3 days per week

Table 9.2 Metabolic Phase Week 1: Microcycle 1

Carry out the first set at an RIR of 3, the second at an RIR of 2, and the final set at an RIR of 1. Rest 30 seconds between sets.

DAY	TARGET MUSCLES	EXERCISES	PAGE
Monday	Total body	Dumbbell incline press (3 sets @ 15-20 reps)	51
		Dumbbell one-arm row (3 sets @ 15-20 reps)	35
		Dumbbell shoulder press (3 sets @ 15-20 reps)	81
		Dumbbell standing biceps curl (3 sets @ 15-20 reps)	92
		Dumbbell overhead triceps extension (3 sets @ 15-20 reps)	104
		Leg press (3 sets @ 15-20 reps)	124
		Lying leg curl (3 sets @ 15-20 reps)	136
		Machine standing calf raise (3 sets @ 15-20 reps)	141
		Bicycle crunch (3 sets @ 15-20 reps)	66
Tuesday	Off		
Wednesday	Total body	Barbell chest press (3 sets @ 20-25 reps)	55
		Lat pull-down (3 sets @ 20-25 reps)	46
		Barbell upright row (3 sets @ 20-25 reps)	90
		Barbell curl (3 sets @ 20-25 reps)	99
		Cable triceps press-down (3 sets @ 20-25 reps)	110
		Barbell back squat (3 sets @ 20-25 reps)	121
		Machine seated leg curl (3 sets @ 20-25 reps)	138
		Machine seated calf raise (3 sets @ 20-25 reps)	140
		Cable rope kneeling crunch (3 sets @ 20-25 reps)	69
Thursday	Off		
Friday	Total body	Machine chest press (3 sets @ 25-30 reps)	58
		Cable seated row (3 sets @ 25-30 reps)	41
		Military press (3 sets @ 25-30 reps)	80
		Cable curl (3 sets @ 25-30 reps)	102
		Skull crusher (3 sets @ 25-30 reps)	106
		Walking lunge (3 sets @ 25-30 reps)	114
		Barbell stiff-legged deadlift (3 sets @ 25-30 reps)	129
		Toe press (3 sets @ 25-30 reps)	139
		Roman chair side crunch (3 sets @ 25-30 reps)	67
Saturday	Off		
Sunday	Off		

Table 9.3   Metabolic Phase Week 2: Microcycle 2

Carry out the first set at an RIR of 3, the second at an RIR of 2, and the final set at an RIR of 1. Rest 30 seconds between supersets.

DAY	TARGET MUSCLES	EXERCISES	PAGE
Monday	Total body	Dumbbell chest press supersetted with cable seated row (3 sets @ 15-20 reps)	**53** and **41**
		Military press supersetted with neutral-grip lat pull-down (3 sets @ 15-20 reps)	**80** and **47**
		Barbell curl supersetted with triceps dip (3 sets @ 15-20 reps)	**99** and **111**
		Leg press supersetted with machine seated leg curl (3 sets @ 15-20 reps)	**124** and **138**
Tuesday	Off		
Wednesday	Total body	Barbell incline press supersetted with barbell reverse-grip bent row (3 sets @ 20-25 reps)	**54** and **37**
		Dumbbell shoulder press supersetted with cross cable lat pull-down (3 sets @ 20-25 reps)	**81** and **50**
		Dumbbell standing biceps curl supersetted with machine skull crusher (3 sets @ 20-25 reps)	**92** and **107**
		Barbell front squat supersetted with dumbbell stiff-legged deadlift (3 sets @ 20-25 reps)	**120** and **130**
Thursday	Off		
Friday	Total body	Barbell decline press supersetted with dumbbell one-arm row (3 sets @ 25-30 reps)	**56** and **35**
		Cable upright row supersetted with lat pull-down (3 sets @ 25-30 reps)	**91** and **46**
		Cable curl supersetted with cable triceps press-down (3 sets @ 25-30 reps)	**102** and **110**
		Walking lunge supersetted with lying leg curl (3 sets @ 25-30 reps)	**114** and **136**
Saturday	Off		
Sunday	Off		

Table 9.4   Metabolic Phase Week 3: Microcycle 3

Carry out the first set at an RIR of 3, the second at an RIR of 2, and the final set at an RIR of 1. Rest as little as possible between exercises during each circuit; rest approximately one to two minutes between circuits.

DAY	TARGET MUSCLES	EXERCISES	PAGE
Monday	Total body	Dumbbell incline press (3 sets @ 15-20 reps)	51
		Dumbbell one-arm row (3 sets @ 15-20 reps)	35
		Dumbbell shoulder press (3 sets @ 15-20 reps)	81
		Dumbbell standing biceps curl (3 sets @ 15-20 reps)	92
		Dumbbell overhead triceps extension (3 sets @ 15-20 reps)	104
		Leg press (3 sets @ 15-20 reps)	124
		Lying leg curl (3 sets @ 15-20 reps)	136
		Machine standing calf raise (3 sets @ 15-20 reps)	141
		Bicycle crunch (3 sets @ 15-20 reps)	66
Tuesday	Off		
Wednesday	Total body	Barbell chest press (3 sets @ 20-25 reps)	55
		Lat pull-down (3 sets @ 20-25 reps)	46
		Barbell upright row (3 sets @ 20-25 reps)	90
		Barbell curl (3 sets @ 20-25 reps)	99
		Cable triceps press-down (3 sets @ 20-25 reps)	110
		Barbell back squat (3 sets @ 20-25 reps)	121
		Machine seated leg curl (3 sets @ 20-25 reps)	138
		Machine seated calf raise (3 sets @ 20-25 reps)	140
		Cable rope kneeling crunch (3 sets @ 20-25 reps)	69
Thursday	Off		
Friday	Total body	Machine chest press (3 sets @ 25-30 reps)	58
		Cable seated row (3 sets @ 25-30 reps)	41
		Military press (3 sets @ 25-30 reps)	80
		Cable curl (3 sets @ 25-30 reps)	102
		Skull crusher (3 sets @ 25-30 reps)	106
		Walking lunge (3 sets @ 25-30 reps)	114
		Barbell stiff-legged deadlift (3 sets @ 25-30 reps)	129
		Toe press (3 sets @ 25-30 reps)	139
		Roman chair side crunch (3 sets @ 25-30 reps)	67
Saturday	Off		
Sunday	Off		

Table 9.5   Metabolic Phase Week 4: Microcycle 4

Perform each set at an RIR of about 4.

DAY	TARGET MUSCLES	EXERCISES	PAGE
Monday	Total body	Dumbbell incline fly (3 sets @ 15-20 reps)	**60**
		Lat pull-down (3 sets @ 15-20 reps)	**46**
		Barbell upright row (3 sets @ 15-20 reps)	**90**
		Bulgarian squat (3 sets @ 15-20 reps)	**123**
		Lying leg curl (3 sets @ 15-20 reps)	**136**
		Machine standing calf raise (3 sets @ 15-20 reps)	**141**
		Plank (3 sets @ 30 sec static hold)	**72**
Tuesday	Off		
Wednesday	Off		
Thursday	Total body	Cable fly (3 sets @ 15-20 reps)	**62**
		Cable seated row (3 sets @ 15-20 reps)	**41**
		Dumbbell lateral raise (3 sets @ 15-20 reps)	**83**
		Dumbbell reverse lunge (3 sets @ 15-20 reps)	**117**
		Machine seated leg curl (3 sets @ 15-20 reps)	**138**
		Toe press (3 sets @ 15-20 reps)	**139**
		Side bridge (3 sets @ 30 sec static hold)	**73**
Friday	Off		
Saturday	Off		
Sunday	Off		

CHAPTER 10

M.A.X. MUSCLE PHASE

The M.A.X. muscle phase is the culmination of the M.A.X. Muscle Plan. As the name implies, this phase is designed to maximize muscle development from both a quantitative (muscle size) and a qualitative (muscle symmetry) standpoint. You'll expend a lot of sweat and effort, but the results will be well worth it—guaranteed!

This phase capitalizes on the results you achieved in the previous phases of the program. Specifically, the strength you gained in the strength phase will facilitate your ability to handle heavier weights—and thus enhance mechanical tension—during hypertrophy training. What's more, the improved metabolic efficiency you achieved in the metabolic phase will allow for increased time under tension (i.e., more reps at a given workload) and heighten your capacity to tolerate greater overall volumes of work. In the M.A.X. muscle phase, you'll capitalize on these adaptations, leveraging them to reach your muscular potential.

PROGRAM PROTOCOL

The M.A.X. muscle phase is an 11- to 12-week mesocycle made up of three distinct training blocks. You'll use moderate-intensity loads (6-12 reps) with moderate rest intervals (1-2 minutes between sets). This combination provides a favorable mix of mechanical tension and metabolic stress that's conducive to maximizing muscle development.

You'll perform multiple sets for each exercise totaling approximately 25-30 sets per session. You'll directly work larger muscle groups (such as the quads, glutes, and back) with a relatively high training volume. Conversely, the muscles of the arms and calves generally receive fewer total direct sets given their function as synergists in many multi-joint exercises.

It's important to note that the volume recommendations herein are merely general guidelines. The total volume performed for each block (the sum of all the sets for every muscle group combined) should be modified based on your individual response. Some lifters do better with relatively lower volumes, whereas others thrive on somewhat higher volumes. Stay in tune with your body (e.g., know signs of fatigue, recovery, and progress) and adjust as needed over time.

Think of this phase as a "specialization cycle" where you focus on bringing up your weak areas with targeted higher amounts of volume. Apportion volume so that more sets are allocated to lagging muscles and fewer to well-developed muscles. Just be sure to stay within your "volume budget," as described in chapter 2, for each block so that a proper balance of stimulus and recovery is maintained.

Also note the long-held belief that larger muscles should be trained first in a session has little scientific credence from a hypertrophy standpoint (5). For best results, exercise order should be prioritized so that lagging muscles are trained early in the workout; you'll be able to exert maximum energy into developing your weak areas when you are fresh and at your best.

Training frequency progressively increases over the course of the meso-cycle to support the cyclical increases in training volumes, ultimately culminating with a "shock phase" designed to bring about short-term over-reaching (see table 10.1 for a schedule). Reduced-frequency deload periods are interspersed throughout the mesocycle to ensure adequate recuperation, with an active recovery period instituted after the final training block. In general, the full effects of supercompensation should manifest about a week or so after you complete an overreaching microcycle, meaning you should realize optimal muscular gains sometime toward the end of the active recovery microcycle.

A core group of multi-joint free weight exercises are kept in constant rotation throughout this phase. Perform these exercises at least once per week to help maintain motor skills. Other exercises, in particular single-joint and machine-based movements, change liberally from one workout to the next to

Table 10.1 Training Frequency Schedule

BLOCK	MICROCYCLE	TRAINING FREQUENCY	DAYS	REGIONS TARGETED
1	1-3	3 days per week	Monday Wednesday Friday	Chest, shoulders, triceps Legs Back, biceps, abdomen
	4	2 days per week (deload)	Monday, Thursday	Total body
2	1-3	4 days per week	Monday, Thursday Tuesday, Friday	Upper body Lower body
	4	2 days per week (deload)	Monday, Thursday	Total body
3	1-2	6 days per week	Monday, Friday Tuesday, Saturday Wednesday, Sunday	Back, chest, abdomen Legs Shoulders, arms
	3	Active recovery		Light aerobic exercise

stimulate the full spectrum of muscle fibers and provide an ongoing, novel stimulus to the neuromuscular system.

It's important to note that the concept of exercise rotation needs to be expanded beyond simply performing an array of exercises for a given muscle; you also need to consider how these movements interact with each other. Basic applied kinesiology principles indicate that certain exercises are complementary, working together to optimize symmetrical muscle development. Factors such as the angle of pull, plane of movement, length–tension relationship, number of joints involved, and other considerations all influence how effectively you work a given muscle. Unfortunately, the vast majority of lifters do not fully comprehend these complexities and continue to haphazardly string together a series of exercises without regard to how they mesh. I have carefully selected the exercises in the sample routines to exemplify how you can work different areas of the target muscles in each training session. In effect, the exercises combine to synergistically develop each target muscle, creating balance both within and between muscle groups; overlap between movements is minimized.

To ensure that you work each muscle to its fullest extent, employ a mix of modalities (free weights, machines, and cables) over the course of the mesocycle. That said, consider the exercises merely as suggestions as to how a hypertrophy-oriented routine can be constructed. As mentioned in chapter 2, there is no such thing as a "must-do" exercise. Thus, feel free to substitute exercises to suit your preferences and equipment availability; just make sure that substitutions take into account the aforementioned kinesiological principles to optimize stimulation of the musculature. It's important that exercises feel good during performance. This allows you to better connect with the movement, strengthening your mind–muscle connection and hence facilitating your ability to get the most out of your efforts.

To enhance the growth response, several advanced training techniques can be incorporated into this phase. These techniques should be limited to a select few sets throughout the training cycle because the fatiguing nature of these techniques increases the potential for overtraining and psychological burnout. As a general guideline, use them on the final set of an exercise or the final set for a given muscle group. Here is an overview of the special techniques to consider using in this phase.

DROP SETS

Drop sets, also known as **strip sets** or **descending sets**, involve performing a set to muscle failure with a given load and then immediately reducing the load and continuing to train until subsequent failure. In other words, you essentially take your sets "beyond failure." This strategy enhances muscle fiber fatigue and metabolic stress. Research is somewhat mixed as to whether drop sets promote an added hypertrophic stimulus to traditional

VARIETY

For the M.A.X. muscle phase, structure exercise selection using a multi-angled, multi-planar, multi-modality approach. As discussed previously, performing an assortment of moves helps stimulate all the fibers in your musculature to elicit maximal muscle growth and symmetry.

When perusing the sample routines in this chapter, you'll note that I provide a wide assortment of exercises that vary from one workout to the next. However, understand that my intention herein is simply to show the potential for incorporating different movements into your routine, not to suggest that every training session must be different from the previous one. That said, you should strive to change at least some of the exercises on a regular basis, as previously described, focusing on more frequent rotation of single-joint and machine-based movements. There is no hard-and-fast rule for how often such changes should be implemented, but a good rule of thumb is to switch things up at least every few weeks. Remember, up to a certain point, variety is the spice of muscle development!

training programs; some studies show a benefit (3), while others don't (1) on a volume-equated basis. That said, there is no evidence that the strategy is detrimental to gains, and at the very least, it can help increase total training volume without adding much extra time to the training session—a favorable risk–reward ratio.

For best results, aim to strip off the weights as quickly as possible; resting more than a few seconds between drop sets diminishes the purported beneficial effects of the technique. Selectorized machines are ideal for this strategy because you only need to move a pin to reduce the load. Dumbbells also work quite well, assuming you can stay close to a rack with a variety of weights lined up for your use. You can perform multiple drops in the same set to elicit even greater levels of fatigue and stress.

ECCENTRIC OVERLOAD

Eccentric overload training (a.k.a. heavy negatives) involves performing eccentric actions using a relatively heavy weight, one that is potentially greater than your concentric 1RM. Research indicates that including heavy negatives in a routine can magnify the growth response and promote region-specific hypertrophy in a given muscle (4). Although the mechanisms are as yet unclear, it likely results from a combination of factors that include greater mechanical tension and possibly heightened localized muscle damage.

Perhaps the easiest application of eccentric overload training is to use a machine where both limbs work dependently to lift a weight. You lift the load concentrically using both limbs, but then lower it using only one leg or arm. For example, in the leg extension, you would extend the legs simultaneously, and when you reach the top portion of the movement, you remove one of your legs from the pad and lower with the other leg. You then alternate between legs on the lowering portion until completion. Alternatively, you can employ this strategy using barbells with supramaximal loads as follows. Load the bar with a weight that is approximately 25 percent heavier than your 1RM for a given exercise. For example, if your maximum bench press is 200 pounds (90.7 kg), use 250 pounds (113.4 kg). Perform an eccentric repetition at a tempo of approximately two to three seconds, making sure to lower the weight in a controlled fashion so that the target muscles are forced to carry out the work. When you reach the bottom portion of the lift, have a spotter help you raise the weight back to the start position. Aim for three to four reps per set. The caveat here is that you must have a spotter; if not, opt for a different modality to carry out the strategy.

LOADED STRETCH

As the name implies, loaded stretch training involves holding a muscle in a stretched position while under load. There is compelling evidence in animal research showing that loaded stretch training can produce massive increases in muscle growth. Research dating back to the late 1980s on attaching loads to the stretched wings of quails (equating to 10-35 percent of each bird's body weight) produced approximately 300 percent gains in muscle mass in just over a month's time (2)! Intriguingly, some of the gains were attributed to muscle hyperplasia (i.e., the formation of new muscle fibers from existing fibers), which generally does not occur from traditional exercise. The kicker here is that the stretch training was maintained for days on end over the study period, limiting the practical relevance of the findings. That said, there is research, albeit limited, indicating that brief periods of loaded stretch may in fact enhance hypertrophy in humans (6, 7).

Although several options exist for employing loaded stretch training, the most effective and efficient approach appears to be integrating the strategy into the interset rest period. In this scenario, you complete a set and then hold the weight in the stretched position for a prescribed period of time. Anecdotally, I've found the sweet spot to be somewhere between 10 and 30 seconds. As a general guideline, stay on the shorter end of the range when using heavier loads and the higher end of the spectrum for lighter loads. The type of exercise (e.g., single versus multi-joint, machine versus free weight, etc.) also affects stretch duration; the more stress on the joint, the less time you should hold the stretch. Importantly, after finishing the loaded stretch, make sure to rest the prescribed amount of time, if not longer, as detailed in table 10.2 on page 192; otherwise, you risk impairing the ability to maintain volume load in the ensuing exercise, which in turn may compromise results.

PROGRAM SPECIFICS

The M.A.X. muscle phase mesocycle allocates training into three blocks that consist of four one-week microcycles. Training volume progressively increases each block so that you achieve a sufficient amount of volume to maximize growth without overtraining. In effect, each block builds on the results achieved in the previous block. Rep range varies using a step-loading model in which deload cycles are interspersed at regular intervals to promote optimal recovery. Rest approximately two minutes between sets for multi-joint exercises and 60 to 90 seconds between sets for single-joint exercises.

Here are the particulars of each block.

BLOCK 1

Block 1 is made up of four one-week microcycles. During the first three microcycles, you'll train on three nonconsecutive days per week (e.g., Monday, Wednesday, and Friday). Training incorporates a three-day push–pull split: You'll work the chest, shoulders, and triceps on day 1; the lower-body musculature on day 2; and the back, biceps, and abs on day 3. You'll perform two to four sets of two to four exercises per muscle group. The loads are carried out using the following step-loading progression.

The first microcycle in block 1 (week 1 of the mesocycle) targets a load corresponding to 10 to 12 repetitions. Your level of effort should correspond to an RIR of 1 or 2 on the initial sets of each exercise, and you should take the last set to the point of concentric muscle failure (RIR of 0).

The second microcycle in block 1 (week 2) targets a load corresponding to 8 to 10 repetitions. Your level of effort should correspond to an RIR of 1 or 2 on the initial sets of each exercise, and you should take the last set to the point of concentric muscle failure (RIR of 0).

The third microcycle in block 1 (week 3) targets a load corresponding to 6 to 8 repetitions. Your level of effort should correspond to an RIR of 1 or 2 on the initial sets of each exercise, and you should take the last set to the point of concentric muscle failure (RIR of 0).

The fourth microcycle in block 1 (week 4) is a deload. You'll train two days per week, allowing 72 hours between sessions (e.g., Monday and Thursday), and follow a total-body routine that works all the major muscle groups during each session. You'll perform one exercise of three sets per muscle group. The rep range will be 15 to 20 repetitions. Sets should not be overly challenging. Aim for an RIR of 4 or so. If you struggle on the last few reps, reduce the weight.

BLOCK 2

Block 2 is made up of four one-week microcycles. During the first three microcycles, you'll train four days per week using a sequence of either two on, one off, two on, two off (e.g., Monday, Tuesday, Thursday, and Friday) or two on, one off, one on, one off, one on, one off (e.g., Monday, Tuesday, Thursday, and Saturday). Training incorporates a two-day split: You'll work the upper body on days 1 and 3 and the lower body on days 2 and 4. Abdominal training is included on the lower-body days. You'll perform three to four sets of one to two exercises per muscle group. Intensity is carried out using the following step-loading progression.

The first microcycle in block 2 (week 5 of the mesocycle) targets a load corresponding to 10 to 12 repetitions. Your level of effort should correspond to an RIR of 1 or 2 on the initial sets of each exercise, and you should take the last set to the point of concentric muscle failure (RIR of 0).

The second microcycle in block 2 (week 6) targets a load corresponding to 8 to 10 repetitions. Your level of effort should correspond to an RIR of 1 or 2 on the initial sets of each exercise, and you should take the last set to the point of concentric muscle failure (RIR of 0).

The third microcycle in block 2 (week 7) targets a load corresponding to 6 to 8 repetitions. Your level of effort should correspond to an RIR of 1 or 2 on the initial sets of each exercise, and you should take the last set to the point of concentric muscle failure (RIR of 0).

The fourth microcycle in block 2 (week 8) is a deload. You'll train two days per week, allowing 72 hours between sessions (e.g., Monday and Thursday), and follow a total-body routine that works all the major muscle groups during each session. You'll perform one exercise of three sets per muscle group. The rep range will be 15 to 20 repetitions. Sets should not be overly challenging; as with the previous deload microcycles, aim for an RIR of about 4.

BLOCK 3

Block 3 is made up of three to four one-week microcycles (two to three training microcycles followed by an active recovery microcycle). If you're a beginner to intermediate lifter, perform two training microcycles; if you're an advanced lifter, consider adding a third training microcycle similar to week 9 or week 10 if you feel sufficiently recovered after the second microcycle.

During each of the training microcycles, you'll work out six days per week using a sequence of three on, one off, three on (i.e., Monday, Tuesday, Wednesday, Friday, Saturday, and Sunday). Training incorporates a three-day, agonist–antagonist split: You'll work the back, chest, and abdominal muscles on days 1 and 4; the lower-body musculature on days 2 and 5; and the shoulders and arms on days 3 and 6. You'll perform two to four sets of two to four exercises per muscle group. Repetitions are carried out using the following progression.

The first microcycle (week 9 of the mesocycle) targets a load corresponding to 10 to 12 repetitions. Your level of effort should correspond to an RIR of 1 or 2 on the initial sets of each exercise, and you should take the last set to the point of concentric muscle failure (RIR of 0).

The second microcycle (week 10) targets a load corresponding to 6 to 8 repetitions. Your level of effort should correspond to an RIR of 1 or 2 on the initial sets of each exercise, and you should take the last set to the point of concentric muscle failure (RIR of 0).

Provided you performed the routine as specified, you should be pretty spent by the end of the M.A.X. muscle phase since its intent is to elicit short-term functional overreaching. Accordingly, after finishing the training microcycles in block 3, you'll engage in a one-week active recovery period to allow for optimal restoration of your body's resources and help prevent overtraining. During this time, perform only light aerobic exercise at a relatively low intensity for 30 to 40 minutes most days of the week. Exercise modalities ideally should incorporate both upper- and lower-body musculature (e.g., elliptical trainers, cross-country ski trainers, jumping jacks) to enhance blood flow throughout the body. Perform no resistance training during this time. Assess how you feel after the first week of active recovery: If you're fresh and vibrant, feel free to get back to lifting; if you're still somewhat fatigued, take an extra week of active recovery. It's better to err on the side of caution and abstain if you have any doubts because restarting too soon can potentially lead to an overtrained state.

Table 10.2 summarizes the M.A.X. muscle phase protocol, and sample routines (tables 10.3 through 10.12) are provided on the subsequent pages. These routines should serve as a basic template for constructing your workouts. As previously noted, modify specific exercises and training volume according to your individual needs and abilities.

Table 10.2   Summary of the Muscle Protocol

TRAINING VARIABLE	PROTOCOL
Repetitions	6-12
Sets	2-4 per exercise
Rest interval	1-2 min
Tempo	Mind–muscle connection
Frequency	3-6 days per week

Table 10.3 M.A.X. Muscle Phase Week 1: Block 1 Microcycle 1

Perform initial sets at an RIR of 1 or 2, and take the last set to the point of concentric muscle failure (RIR of 0).

DAY	TARGET MUSCLES	EXERCISES	PAGE
Monday	Chest, shoulders, triceps	Barbell incline press (4 sets @ 10-12 reps)	54
		Dumbbell chest press (3 sets @ 10-12 reps)	53
		Pec deck fly (3 sets @ 10-12 reps)	61
		Military press (4 sets @ 10-12 reps)	80
		Cable lateral raise (3 sets @ 10-12 reps)	85
		Machine rear delt fly (3 sets @ 10-12 reps)	87
		Dumbbell overhead triceps extension (3 sets @ 10-12 reps)	104
		Skull crusher (2 sets @ 10-12 reps)	106
		Machine triceps dip (2 sets @ 10-12 reps)	112
Tuesday	Off		
Wednesday	Legs	Barbell back squat (4 sets @ 10-12 reps)	121
		Dumbbell reverse lunge (4 sets @ 10-12 reps)	117
		Leg extension (3 sets @ 10-12 reps)	134
		Barbell stiff-legged deadlift (4 sets @ 10-12 reps)	129
		Lying leg curl (4 sets @ 10-12 reps)	136
		Machine seated calf raise (4 sets @ 10-12 reps)	140
		Machine standing calf raise (3 sets @ 10-12 reps)	141
Thursday	Off		
Friday	Back, biceps, abdomen	Lat pull-down (4 sets @ 10-12 reps)	46
		Cable seated row (4 sets @ 10-12 reps)	41
		Dumbbell pullover (4 sets @ 10-12 reps)	34
		Barbell curl (3 sets @ 10-12 reps)	99
		Cable rope hammer curl (2 sets @ 10-12 reps)	101
		Concentration curl (2 sets @ 10-12 reps)	97
		Stability ball abdominal crunch (3 sets @ 10-12 reps)	68
		Reverse crunch (3 sets @ 10-12 reps)	65
		Russian twist (2 sets @ 10-12 reps)	75
Saturday	Off		
Sunday	Off		

Table 10.4   M.A.X. Muscle Phase Week 2: Block 1 Microcycle 2

Perform initial sets at an RIR of 1 or 2, and take the last set to the point of concentric muscle failure (RIR of 0).

DAY	TARGET MUSCLES	EXERCISES	PAGE
Monday	Chest, shoulders, triceps	Dumbbell incline press (4 sets @ 8-10 reps)	51
		Barbell decline press (3 sets @ 8-10 reps)	56
		Dumbbell flat fly (3 sets @ 8-10 reps)	59
		Dumbbell shoulder press (4 sets @ 8-10 reps)	81
		Cable upright row (3 sets @ 8-10 reps)	91
		Dumbbell bent reverse fly (3 sets @ 8-10 reps)	86
		Cable rope overhead triceps extension (2 sets @ 8-10 reps)	105
		Cable triceps press-down (2 sets @ 8-10 reps)	110
		Triceps dip (2 sets @ 8-10 reps)	111
Tuesday	Off		
Wednesday	Legs	Barbell front squat (4 sets @ 8-10 reps)	120
		Dumbbell step-up (4 sets @ 8-10 reps)	119
		Sissy squat (3 sets @ 8-10 reps)	128
		Good morning (4 sets @ 8-10 reps)	127
		Machine seated leg curl (3 sets @ 8-10 reps)	138
		Toe press (4 sets @ 8-10 reps)	139
		Machine seated calf raise (3 sets @ 8-10 reps)	140
Thursday	Off		
Friday	Back, biceps, abdomen	Cross cable lat pull-down (4 sets @ 8-10 reps)	50
		Dumbbell one-arm row (4 sets @ 8-10 reps)	35
		Cable straight-arm lat pull-down (3 sets @ 8-10 reps)	49
		Dumbbell incline biceps curl (3 sets @ 8-10 reps)	93
		Barbell preacher curl (3 sets @ 8-10 reps)	95
		Hanging knee raise (3 sets @ 8-10 reps)	74
		Cable wood chop (3 sets @ 8-10 reps)	77
Saturday	Off		
Sunday	Off		

Table 10.5   M.A.X. Muscle Phase Week 3: Block 1 Microcycle 3

Perform initial sets at an RIR of 1 or 2, and take the last set to the point of concentric muscle failure (RIR of 0).

DAY	TARGET MUSCLES	EXERCISES	PAGE
Monday	Chest, shoulders, triceps	Machine chest press (4 sets @ 6-8 reps)	58
		Dumbbell incline press (4 sets @ 6-8 reps)	51
		Cable fly (3 sets @ 6-8 reps)	62
		Machine shoulder press (4 sets @ 6-8 reps)	82
		Dumbbell lateral raise (3 sets @ 6-8 reps)	83
		Cable reverse fly (3 sets @ 6-8 reps)	88
		Machine skull crusher (3 sets @ 6-8 reps)	107
		Dumbbell overhead triceps extension (2 sets @ 6-8 reps)	104
		Cable triceps kickback (2 sets @ 6-8 reps)	109
Tuesday	Off		
Wednesday	Legs	Leg press (4 sets @ 6-8 reps)	124
		Dumbbell lunge (4 sets @ 6-8 reps)	116
		Unilateral leg extension (3 sets @ 6-8 reps)	135
		Barbell hip thrust (4 sets @ 6-8 reps)	126
		Machine kneeling leg curl (4 sets @ 6-8 reps)	137
		Machine seated calf raise (4 sets @ 6-8 reps)	140
		Machine standing calf raise (4 sets @ 6-8 reps)	141
Thursday	Off		
Friday	Back, biceps, abdomen	Chin-up (4 sets @ 6-8 reps)	44
		Machine wide-grip seated row (4 sets @ 6-8 reps)	40
		Cable one-arm standing low row (4 sets @ 6-8 reps)	43
		Cable one-arm curl (3 sets @ 6-8 reps)	103
		Dumbbell standing hammer curl (2 sets @ 6-8 reps)	98
		Machine preacher curl (2 sets @ 6-8 reps)	96
		Toe touch (3 sets @ 6-8 reps)	71
		Cable side bend (2 sets @ 6-8 reps)	76
		Side bridge (2 sets @ 30 sec static hold)	73
Saturday	Off		
Sunday	Off		

Table 10.6   M.A.X. Muscle Phase Week 4: Block 1 Microcycle 4

Perform all exercises at an RIR of approximately 4.

DAY	TARGET MUSCLES	EXERCISES	PAGE
Monday	Total body	Barbell incline press (3 sets @ 15-20 reps)	54
		Lat pull-down (3 sets @ 15-20 reps)	46
		Barbell upright row (3 sets @ 15-20 reps)	90
		Barbell curl (3 sets @ 15-20 reps)	99
		Skull crusher (3 sets @ 15-20 reps)	106
		Barbell back squat (3 sets @ 15-20 reps)	121
		Lying leg curl (3 sets @ 15-20 reps)	136
		Machine standing calf raise (3 sets @ 15-20 reps)	141
		Plank (3 sets @ 30 sec static hold)	72
Tuesday	Off		
Wednesday	Off		
Thursday	Total body	Dumbbell chest press (3 sets @ 15-20 reps)	53
		Barbell overhand bent row (3 sets @ 15-20 reps)	38
		Military press (3 sets @ 15-20 reps)	80
		Dumbbell preacher curl (3 sets @ 15-20 reps)	94
		Cable triceps press-down (3 sets @ 15-20 reps)	110
		Dumbbell reverse lunge (3 sets @ 15-20 reps)	117
		Cable glute kickback (3 sets @ 15-20 reps)	131
		Toe press (3 sets @ 15-20 reps)	139
		Side bridge (3 sets @ 30 sec static hold)	73
Friday	Off		
Saturday	Off		
Sunday	Off		

Table 10.7   M.A.X. Muscle Phase Week 5: Block 2 Microcycle 1

Perform initial sets at an RIR of 1 or 2, and take the last set to the point of concentric muscle failure (RIR of 0).

DAY	TARGET MUSCLES	EXERCISES	PAGE
Monday	Upper body	Barbell chest press (4 sets @ 10-12 reps)	55
		Dumbbell incline fly (3 sets @ 10-12 reps)	60
		Reverse-grip lat pull-down (4 sets @ 10-12 reps)	48
		Cable wide-grip seated row (3 sets @ 10-12 reps)	42
		Dumbbell shoulder press (4 sets @ 10-12 reps)	81
		Cable lateral raise (3 sets @ 10-12 reps)	85
		Barbell drag curl (4 sets @ 10-12 reps)	100
		Dumbbell overhead triceps extension (4 sets @ 10-12 reps)	104
Tuesday	Lower body	Barbell split squat (4 sets @ 10-12 reps)	122
		Leg extension (4 sets @ 10-12 reps)	134
		Barbell stiff-legged deadlift (4 sets @ 10-12 reps)	129
		Lying leg curl (3 sets @ 10-12 reps)	136
		Machine standing calf raise (3 sets @ 10-12 reps)	141
		Machine seated calf raise (3 sets @ 10-12 reps)	140
		Barbell rollout (4 sets @ 10-12 reps)	78
		Cable rope kneeling twisting crunch (3 sets @ 10-12 reps)	70
Wednesday	Off		
Thursday	Upper body	Machine incline press (4 sets @ 10-12 reps)	57
		Pec deck fly (3 sets @ 10-12 reps)	61
		Pull-up (4 sets @ 10-12 reps)	45
		T-bar row (3 sets @ 10-12 reps)	36
		Machine shoulder press (4 sets @ 10-12 reps)	82
		Cable kneeling reverse fly (3 sets @ 10-12 reps)	89
		Dumbbell standing biceps curl (4 sets @ 10-12 reps)	92
		Dumbbell triceps kickback (4 sets @ 10-12 reps)	108
Friday	Lower body	Leg press (4 sets @ 10-12 reps)	124
		Dumbbell side lunge (4 sets @ 10-12 reps)	118
		Hyperextension (4 sets @ 10-12 reps)	132
		Machine seated leg curl (4 sets @ 10-12 reps)	138
		Machine seated calf raise (3 sets @ 10-12 reps)	140
		Toe press (3 sets @ 10-12 reps)	139
		Cable rope kneeling crunch (3 sets @ 10-12 reps)	69
		Cable wood chop (3 sets @ 10-12 reps)	77
Saturday	Off		
Sunday	Off		

Table 10.8   M.A.X. Muscle Phase Week 6: Block 2 Microcycle 2

Perform initial sets at an RIR of 1 or 2, and take the last set to the point of concentric muscle failure (RIR of 0).

DAY	TARGET MUSCLES	EXERCISES	PAGE
Monday	Upper body	Dumbbell incline press (4 sets @ 8-10 reps)	51
		Chest dip (3 sets @ 8-10 reps)	63
		Cross cable lat pull-down (4 sets @ 8-10 reps)	50
		Dumbbell pullover (3 sets @ 8-10 reps)	34
		Cable upright row (4 sets @ 8-10 reps)	91
		Dumbbell bent reverse fly (3 sets @ 8-10 reps)	86
		Dumbbell standing hammer curl (4 sets @ 8-10 reps)	98
		Cable rope overhead triceps extension (4 sets @ 8-10 reps)	105
Tuesday	Lower body	Barbell front squat (4 sets @ 8-10 reps)	120
		Sissy squat (4 sets @ 8-10 reps)	128
		Good morning (4 sets @ 8-10 reps)	127
		Machine kneeling leg curl (3 sets @ 8-10 reps)	137
		Machine standing calf raise (3 sets @ 8-10 reps)	141
		Machine seated calf raise (3 sets @ 8-10 reps)	140
		Cable rope kneeling crunch (4 sets @ 8-10 reps)	69
		Roman chair side crunch (3 sets @ 8-10 reps)	67
Wednesday	Off		
Thursday	Upper body	Barbell decline press (4 sets @ 8-10 reps)	56
		Cable fly (3 sets @ 8-10 reps)	62
		Lat pull-down (4 sets @ 8-10 reps)	46
		Barbell reverse-grip bent row (3 sets @ 8-10 reps)	37
		Machine shoulder press (4 sets @ 8-10 reps)	82
		Cable lateral raise (3 sets @ 8-10 reps)	85
		Concentration curl (4 sets @ 8-10 reps)	97
		Machine triceps dip (4 sets @ 8-10 reps)	112
Friday	Lower body	Barbell lunge (4 sets @ 8-10 reps)	115
		Dumbbell step-up (4 sets @ 8-10 reps)	119
		Reverse hyperextension (3 sets @ 8-10 reps)	133
		Lying leg curl (4 sets @ 8-10 reps)	136
		Machine seated calf raise (3 sets @ 8-10 reps)	140
		Machine standing calf raise (3 sets @ 8-10 reps)	141
		Reverse crunch (4 sets @ 8-10 reps)	65
		Russian twist (3 sets @ 8-10 reps)	75
Saturday	Off		
Sunday	Off		

Table 10.9   M.A.X. Muscle Phase Week 7: Block 2 Microcycle 3

Perform initial sets at an RIR of 1 or 2, and take the last set to the point of concentric muscle failure (RIR of 0).

DAY	TARGET MUSCLES	EXERCISES	PAGE
Monday	Upper body	Barbell incline press (4 sets @ 6-8 reps)	54
		Dumbbell flat fly (3 sets @ 6-8 reps)	59
		Chin-up (4 sets @ 6-8 reps)	44
		Machine close-grip seated row (3 sets @ 6-8 reps)	39
		Military press (4 sets @ 6-8 reps)	80
		Machine lateral raise (3 sets @ 6-8 reps)	84
		Cable curl (4 sets @ 6-8 reps)	102
		Cable triceps press-down (4 sets @ 6-8 reps)	110
Tuesday	Lower body	Bulgarian squat (4 sets @ 6-8 reps)	123
		Barbell split squat (4 sets @ 6-8 reps)	122
		Cable glute kickback (4 sets @ 6-8 reps)	131
		Machine seated leg curl (4 sets @ 6-8 reps)	138
		Toe press (3 sets @ 6-8 reps)	139
		Machine seated calf raise (3 sets @ 6-8 reps)	140
		Hanging knee raise (3 sets @ 6-8 reps)	74
Wednesday	Off		
Thursday	Upper body	Dumbbell chest press (4 sets @ 6-8 reps)	53
		Pec deck fly (3 sets @ 6-8 reps)	61
		Lat pull-down (4 sets @ 6-8 reps)	46
		Dumbbell one-arm row (3 sets @ 6-8 reps)	35
		Dumbbell shoulder press (4 sets @ 6-8 reps)	81
		Dumbbell lateral raise (3 sets @ 6-8 reps)	83
		Dumbbell incline biceps curl (4 sets @ 6-8 reps)	93
		Skull crusher (4 sets @ 6-8 reps)	106
Friday	Lower body	Dumbbell reverse lunge (4 sets @ 6-8 reps)	117
		Unilateral leg extension (4 sets @ 6-8 reps)	135
		Dumbbell stiff-legged deadlift (4 sets @ 6-8 reps)	130
		Machine kneeling leg curl (4 sets @ 6-8 reps)	137
		Machine standing calf raise (3 sets @ 6-8 reps)	141
		Machine seated calf raise (3 sets @ 6-8 reps)	140
		Toe touch (3 sets @ 6-8 reps)	71
		Cable side bend (3 sets @ 6-8 reps)	76
Saturday	Off		
Sunday	Off		

Table 10.10   M.A.X. Muscle Phase Week 8: Block 2 Microcycle 4

Perform all exercises at an RIR of approximately 4.

DAY	TARGET MUSCLES	EXERCISES	PAGE
Monday	Total body	Barbell chest press (3 sets @ 15-20 reps)	55
		Machine close-grip seated row (3 sets @ 15-20 reps)	39
		Military press (3 sets @ 15-20 reps)	80
		Barbell preacher curl (3 sets @ 15-20 reps)	95
		Dumbbell overhead triceps extension (3 sets @ 15-20 reps)	104
		Barbell front squat (3 sets @ 15-20 reps)	120
		Good morning (3 sets @ 15-20 reps)	127
		Machine standing calf raise (3 sets @ 15-20 reps)	141
		Plank (3 sets @ 30 sec static hold)	72
Tuesday	Off		
Wednesday	Off		
Thursday	Total body	Dumbbell incline fly (3 sets @ 15-20 reps)	60
		Cross cable lat pull-down (3 sets @ 15-20 reps)	50
		Machine shoulder press (3 sets @ 15-20 reps)	82
		Cable rope hammer curl (3 sets @ 15-20 reps)	101
		Cable triceps kickback (3 sets @ 15-20 reps)	109
		Dumbbell lunge (3 sets @ 15-20 reps)	116
		Lying leg curl (3 sets @ 15-20 reps)	136
		Toe press (3 sets @ 15-20 reps)	139
		Side bridge (3 sets @ 30 sec static hold)	73
Friday	Off		
Saturday	Off		
Sunday	Off		

Table 10.11 M.A.X. Muscle Phase Week 9: Block 3 Microcycle 1

Perform initial sets at an RIR of 1 or 2, and take the last set to the point of concentric muscle failure (RIR of 0).

DAY	TARGET MUSCLES	EXERCISES	PAGE
Monday	Back, chest, abdomen	Lat pull-down (4 sets @ 10-12 reps)	46
		Dumbbell one-arm row (3 sets @ 10-12 reps)	35
		Dumbbell pullover (4 sets @ 10-12 reps)	34
		Barbell incline press (4 sets @ 10-12 reps)	54
		Dumbbell decline press (3 sets @ 10-12 reps)	52
		Cable fly (3 sets @ 10-12 reps)	62
		Stability ball abdominal crunch (3 sets @ 10-12 reps)	68
		Russian twist (3 sets @ 10-12 reps)	75
Tuesday	Legs	Barbell back squat (4 sets @ 10-12 reps)	121
		Dumbbell side lunge (4 sets @ 10-12 reps)	118
		Sissy squat (3 sets @ 10-12 reps)	128
		Barbell stiff-legged deadlift (4 sets @ 10-12 reps)	129
		Machine seated leg curl (3 sets @ 10-12 reps)	138
		Cable glute kickback (3 sets @ 10-12 reps)	131
		Machine standing calf raise (4 sets @ 10-12 reps)	141
		Machine seated calf raise (3 sets @ 10-12 reps)	140
Wednesday	Shoulders, arms	Military press (4 sets @ 10-12 reps)	80
		Machine lateral raise (4 sets @ 10-12 reps)	84
		Machine rear delt fly (4 sets @ 10-12 reps)	87
		Cable rope overhead triceps extension (3 sets @ 10-12 reps)	105
		Skull crusher (2 sets @ 10-12 reps)	106
		Dumbbell triceps kickback (2 sets @ 10-12 reps)	108
		Cable rope hammer curl (3 sets @ 10-12 reps)	101
		Barbell drag curl (2 sets @ 10-12 reps)	100
		Dumbbell incline biceps curl (2 sets @ 10-12 reps)	93
Thursday	Off		

(continued)

Table 10.11 M.A.X. Muscle Phase Week 9: Block 3 Microcycle 1 *(continued)*

DAY	TARGET MUSCLES	EXERCISES	PAGE
Friday	Back, chest, abdomen	Chin-up (4 sets @ 10-12 reps)	44
		Cable seated row (4 sets @ 10-12 reps)	41
		Cable straight-arm lat pull-down (3 sets @ 10-12 reps)	49
		Dumbbell incline press (4 sets @ 10-12 reps)	51
		Barbell chest press (4 sets @ 10-12 reps)	55
		Pec deck fly (3 sets @ 10-12 reps)	61
		Cable rope kneeling crunch (4 sets @ 10-12 reps)	69
		Hanging knee raise (3 sets @ 10-12 reps)	74
Saturday	Legs	Barbell front squat (4 sets @ 10-12 reps)	120
		Dumbbell reverse lunge (4 sets @ 10-12 reps)	117
		Leg extension (3 sets @ 10-12 reps)	134
		Barbell hip thrust (4 sets @ 10-12 reps)	126
		Cable glute kickback (4 sets @ 10-12 reps)	131
		Machine kneeling leg curl (3 sets @ 10-12 reps)	137
		Machine standing calf raise (4 sets @ 10-12 reps)	141
		Machine seated calf raise (3 sets @ 10-12 reps)	140
Sunday	Shoulders, arms	Dumbbell shoulder press (4 sets @ 10-12 reps)	81
		Cable lateral raise (3 sets @ 10-12 reps)	85
		Machine rear delt fly (3 sets @ 10-12 reps)	87
		Cable triceps press-down (3 sets @ 10-12 reps)	110
		Machine skull crusher (2 sets @ 10-12 reps)	107
		Triceps dip (2 sets @ 10-12 reps)	111
		Dumbbell incline biceps curl (3 sets @ 10-12 reps)	93
		Concentration curl (2 sets @ 10-12 reps)	97
		Dumbbell standing hammer curl (2 sets @ 10-12 reps)	98

Table 10.12   M.A.X. Muscle Phase Week 10: Block 3 Microcycle 2

Perform initial sets at an RIR of 1 or 2, and take the last set to the point of concentric muscle failure (RIR of 0).

DAY	TARGET MUSCLES	EXERCISES	PAGE
Monday	Back, chest, abdomen	Cross cable lat pull-down (4 sets @ 6-8 reps)	50
		Reverse-grip lat pull-down (4 sets @ 6-8 reps)	48
		Machine wide-grip seated row (3 sets @ 6-8 reps)	40
		Barbell chest press (4 sets @ 6-8 reps)	55
		Dumbbell incline press (4 sets @ 6-8 reps)	51
		Pec deck fly (3 sets @ 6-8 reps)	61
		Reverse crunch (4 sets @ 6-8 reps)	65
		Cable wood chop (3 sets @ 6-8 reps)	77
Tuesday	Legs	Leg press (4 sets @ 6-8 reps)	124
		Dumbbell lunge (4 sets @ 6-8 reps)	116
		Unilateral leg extension (3 sets @ 6-8 reps)	135
		Good morning (4 sets @ 6-8 reps)	127
		Lying leg curl (4 sets @ 6-8 reps)	136
		Machine seated calf raise (4 sets @ 6-8 reps)	140
		Machine standing calf raise (3 sets @ 6-8 reps)	141
Wednesday	Shoulders, arms	Military press (4 sets @ 6-8 reps)	80
		Dumbbell lateral raise (4 sets @ 6-8 reps)	83
		Cable reverse fly (3 sets @ 6-8 reps)	88
		Cable rope overhead triceps extension (4 sets @ 6-8 reps)	105
		Cable triceps kickback (3 sets @ 6-8 reps)	109
		Barbell preacher curl (4 sets @ 6-8 reps)	95
		Dumbbell standing biceps curl (3 sets @ 6-8 reps)	92
Thursday	Off		
Friday	Back, chest, abdomen	Neutral-grip lat pull-down (4 sets @ 6-8 reps)	47
		Dumbbell one-arm row (4 sets @ 6-8 reps)	35
		Dumbbell pullover (3 sets @ 6-8 reps)	34
		Dumbbell incline press (4 sets @ 6-8 reps)	51
		Barbell decline press (4 sets @ 6-8 reps)	56
		Cable fly (3 sets @ 6-8 reps)	62
		Cable rope kneeling twisting crunch (4 sets @ 6-8 reps)	70
		Roman chair side crunch (3 sets @ 6-8 reps)	67

(continued)

Table 10.12 M.A.X. Muscle Phase Week 10: Block 3 Microcycle 2 *(continued)*

DAY	TARGET MUSCLES	EXERCISES	PAGE
Saturday	Legs	Barbell back squat (4 sets @ 6-8 reps)	121
		Dumbbell step-up (4 sets @ 6-8 reps)	119
		Sissy squat (4 sets @ 6-8 reps)	128
		Good morning (4 sets @ 6-8 reps)	127
		Lying leg curl (4 sets @ 6-8 reps)	136
		Machine seated calf raise (4 sets @ 6-8 reps)	140
		Machine standing calf raise (3 sets @ 6-8 reps)	141
Sunday	Shoulders, arms	Military press (4 sets @ 6-8 reps)	80
		Cable upright row (4 sets @ 6-8 reps)	91
		Machine rear delt fly (4 sets @ 6-8 reps)	87
		Cable triceps press-down (4 sets @ 6-8 reps)	110
		Skull crusher (3 sets @ 6-8 reps)	106
		Cable curl (4 sets @ 6-8 reps)	102
		Concentration curl (3 sets @ 6-8 reps)	97

M.A.X. NUTRITION

Training and nutrition go hand in hand from a hypertrophy standpoint. Although we can quibble over the relative importance of these two components to body composition, one thing is certain: Proper nutrition is vital to maximizing muscle development. You must eat properly to grow!

Because it would take an entire book to detail the complexities of nutrition science as it pertains to muscle building, this chapter covers only the basics. What follows is an overview of the primary dietary factors that affect muscle development—namely, calories and macronutrients (protein, carbohydrate, and fat).

Theories about how many calories and which foods to consume in which quantities abound. Unfortunately, many are based on anecdotes, myths, and misinterpretations of research. The information presented herein will help you determine what to eat and in what quantities as well as explain how and why your nutritional choices make a difference. Note that all recommendations that are based on body weight should be interpreted as "lean" weight, defined herein as a weight corresponding to approximately 10 percent body fat for a male and 20 percent body fat for a female because this is consistent with findings from the research.

NUTRITIONAL RECOMMENDATIONS

Consider my dietary recommendations as flexible guidelines for creating a customized muscle-building diet rather than unyielding nutritional dogma. Although these recommendations are grounded in science, take into account your own preferences, goals, and experiences; this is the essence of evidence-based practice. There is a great deal of variance in how people respond to different foods. Some trial and error, therefore, is required to determine your optimal caloric intake and macronutrient ratios. Be prepared to experiment until you get it right. Moreover, a nutritional regimen is only as good as your desire to continue eating in this fashion. Adherence is paramount; if you can't stick to a diet, it's essentially worthless.

CALORIES

As a general rule, you need to consume a surplus of calories (a.k.a. energy) to achieve optimal increases in muscle mass. Although it's possible to gain muscle while losing body fat—a phenomenon called **body recomposition**—the extent of muscular increases will be limited and contingent on several factors (see the Can You Simultaneously Gain Muscle and Lose Body Fat? sidebar in this chapter). A calorie surplus facilitates muscle building by supporting the demands of intensive training. This not only includes exercise performance but also the sustenance of post-exercise elevations in energy expenditure (in particular, the breakdown and synthesis of body proteins) as well as the energetic cost of maintaining additional muscle mass (3).

The theoretical benefit of a caloric surplus for gaining mass is consistent with the first law of thermodynamics, which states that energy can be neither created nor destroyed, only changed from one form to another. From a nutritional standpoint, the first law of thermodynamics can be expressed by the following equation:

$$\text{calories in} - \text{calories out} = \text{change in body mass}$$

CAN YOU SIMULTANEOUSLY GAIN MUSCLE AND LOSE BODY FAT?

A majority of lifters seek to gain muscle while losing body fat—a concept popularly known as body recomposition. Without question, body recomposition is an achievable goal. It's been well documented in the literature (11, 35), and I've seen it occur frequently throughout the course of my own research efforts.

The extent to which you can accomplish body recomposition depends on two primary factors: initial body fat level and training status. Higher amounts of body fat facilitate the ability to achieve recomposition; the leaner you get, the harder it is to lose fat while building muscle. Similarly, newbies to lifting (or those who have taken an extended time off from training) can add muscle relatively easily while cutting; as you gain training experience, this feat becomes increasingly more difficult. Being both relatively lean and well-trained further compounds matters; don't expect to have much luck recomping in this case.

Importantly, while body recomposition is indeed possible, you cannot maximize hypertrophic gains under these circumstances because losing body fat requires maintaining a caloric deficit. Even moderate hypocaloric conditions (20 percent below maintenance requirements) for short time periods blunt muscle protein synthesis and anabolic signaling (44). Conceivably this is due to heightened activation of AMPK, a catabolic enzyme that acts as an energy sensor; when caloric intake is low, AMPK activity ramps up and antagonizes anabolic processes in an attempt to conserve energy (12). Bottom line: If your goal is to optimize your hypertrophic potential, you must focus on eating in an energy surplus and accept that you'll gain some extra body fat in the process.

The ramifications of this equation are clear: When you take in more calories than you expend, the excess energy is stored in the form of body mass. However, whether the additional mass is gained as muscle or fat depends on a host of diet- and training-related factors.

Old-school mass-gaining regimens consisted of alternating cycles of bulking and cutting. During the bulking cycles, lifters would scarf down everything imaginable, paying little heed to the types and quantities of foods consumed—the so-called "dirty bulk." Triple cheeseburgers, fries, ice cream, cookies . . . the more calorically rich the food, the better. This unfettered gluttony was then followed by a period of extreme dieting in which the lifters would cut calories to a bare minimum in an effort to lean out. In a perfect world, the strategy would culminate in a huge, shredded physique.

Unfortunately, we don't live in a perfect world.

Sure, the bulking-and-cutting approach significantly helps to increase body mass. I know of a few pro bodybuilders who put on upward of 100 pounds (45 kg) in the bulking phase. There's one little problem with this outcome, though: A large percentage of the weight gain is stored in the form of body fat. Unless you plan to compete as a sumo wrestler, that's far too much. In this scenario, it can take up to a year or more to diet down to an acceptable level of body fat. Worse, hard-earned muscle is inevitably sacrificed in the dieting process. You're lucky to hold on to half of your muscular gains by the time you're lean. It's a poor cost–benefit ratio.

Of even greater concern is that the bulking-and-cutting approach is detrimental to long-term body composition. This appears to be a function of your biological set point. Simply stated, set point is the body's way of physiologically regulating your weight. Through various processes, your body makes a coordinated effort to adjust the intake and expenditure of energy so that a specified amount of fat stores is maintained. Any attempt to deviate from this predetermined level is actively resisted.

As you may imagine, chronic dieting is perceived as a threat to your energy reserves. Accordingly, your body continually trains itself to survive on fewer and fewer calories during each cycle of yo-yo dieting. In an attempt to maintain homeostasis, it alters various hormonal and enzymatic processes; in certain cases, these alterations can be difficult to reverse. Negative effects are fueled by a concomitant loss of lean mass during extreme dieting (i.e., the fat overshooting hypothesis) (25) and an increase not only in the size of fat cells but also their number (adipocyte hyperplasia) when excess calories are subsequently overconsumed (58). The upshot is that your biological set point is reset to a higher level (41), resulting in a predisposition to retain higher levels of body fat in future diet cycles.

The key to a successful muscle-building diet is to keep calories in a range that promotes the development of lean mass while minimizing the accretion of body fat—a.k.a. a "clean bulk." Of note: Training experience can influence the effects of a caloric surplus on body composition. Those with limited training experience are generally able to put on more lean mass without gaining substantial amounts of body fat when consuming a large surplus (50). Alternatively, experienced lifters tend to gain fat more easily when calories are substantially increased above maintenance (15, 46). A gain of about 1 pound (0.5 kg) of lean mass per week can be considered the upper limit of what most can expect to attain without substantially fattening up in the process. For those who have several years of training experience, a gain of about 0.5 pound (0.25 kg) of lean mass per week is probably more realistic, and those who are very well-trained (e.g., competitive bodybuilders) can expect to achieve even slower gains.

So how many calories should you consume to achieve lean gains? As a general guideline, a surplus of 500-1,000 calories a day is a good starting point for newbies. Alternatively, those who've been lifting for a while should aim for a smaller daily surplus of about 250-500 calories (3). These values amount to an increase of approximately 20-40 percent above maintenance requirements for novice trainees and approximately 10-20 percent for more experienced lifters.

You can estimate your energy requirements using various formulas. Although a number of alternatives exist, a particularly good option is the Mifflin-St Jeor equation, which has been shown to be among the most accurate predictive models (37). Just do a web-based search for "Mifflin-St Jeor" and you'll find links to numerous online calculators that use this equation; simply plug in a few numbers and get an instant estimate of caloric maintenance needs. Once you have determined your maintenance requirements, add in the additional calories per the aforementioned recommendations to obtain your suggested daily caloric starting point. Note that the values obtained from formulas are merely estimates of how many calories you require; the actual number ultimately involves a host of genetic and lifestyle factors. The only way to truly gauge actual requirements is via sophisticated metabolic testing, which most people do not have access to. Moreover, there inevitably will be large interindividual differences as to how caloric intake affects the composition of gains in body mass. Thus, it's essential that you closely monitor your weight and make as-needed adjustments in the number of calories consumed. If possible, have your body composition assessed on a regular basis, perhaps once a month or so, by a competent professional. Skinfolds and circumference measures are a good, inexpensive combination in this regard, helping you to determine whether you're making appropriate progress and hence best guide decision-making.

It's essential to approach the process of individualizing caloric consumption in a systematic manner. Do so conservatively, making relatively small caloric adjustments based on progress. I like to use the rule of 100. Start off by consuming your target caloric intake, as estimated by a validated formula (e.g., Mifflin-St Jeor), for a couple of weeks. If you aren't gaining enough mass, increase your intake by an additional 100 calories per day. If, on the other hand, you are gaining too much fat, cut back intake by 100 calories per day. Evaluate your progress after another week or two and continue tweaking in 100-calorie increments as needed. Making these adjustments in a controlled fashion will allow you to fine-tune your diet so that you can optimize the ratio of muscle gains to fat gains.

For best results, track your food consumption on a daily basis. I've found that most people tend to be oblivious to the foods they eat, particularly the quantities. Food plays a huge role in our lives and can be abundant in society. It's often a revelation when a person is forced to track intake; you realize all the times you eat without thinking. Instead of old-school food diaries, you can use a variety of smart apps to make the tracking process relatively simple. Some apps even have the ability to scan food labels. The strategy involves a minimal time investment that can pay big dividends in your gains. If you're serious about getting the most out of your efforts, tracking your intake is a worthy endeavor.

PROTEIN

From a muscle-building perspective, protein can be considered the king of all nutrients. The amino acids in dietary protein sources are the building blocks of muscle tissue, and their presence is required for anabolic signaling pathways to carry out protein synthesis.

Amino acids are divided into two basic categories: essential and nonessential. The essential amino acids (leucine, tryptophan, lysine, methionine, phenyl-alanine, threonine, valine, histidine, and isoleucine) are the most nutritionally significant. The body cannot manufacture these amino acids; therefore, you must obtain them from the foods in your diet. A dietary shortage in even one of the essential amino acids is enough to impair your muscle development.

Protein status in the body is commonly determined by nitrogen balance. A negative nitrogen balance means that your body is breaking down proteins at a greater rate than it is synthesizing them, a positive nitrogen balance means that your body is creating new proteins faster than it is breaking them down, and a stable nitrogen balance means that protein degradation and protein synthesis are in equilibrium.

To build muscle, you need to be in a positive nitrogen balance over time (protein synthesis must exceed protein breakdown). This requires adhering to a protein-rich diet. If your intake of protein is insufficient to make up for what you lose, cellular function is compromised, and muscle development suffers. Only by consuming protein in excess of losses can you promote anabolism and enhance muscle development.

The recommended dietary allowance (RDA) for protein is equal to a little less than 0.4 gram of protein per pound of body weight per day (0.8 g/kg). Not a heck of a lot. One not-so-little caveat: The RDA bases protein require-ments on the needs of the average couch potato. Although this is fine if you aspire to be an average couch potato, it has little relevance if your goal is to maximize muscle development.

Studies indicate that people involved in serious resistance training programs require a protein intake of about 0.75-1 gram per pound (1.6-2.2 g/kg) of body weight to promote anabolism (6). My general recommendation is to err on the high side of the guidelines and consume approximately 1 gram of protein per pound of body weight. For example, if you weigh 200 pounds (91 kg), protein intake should equal approximately 200 grams per day. This provides a margin of safety, ensuring that you remain in a positive nitrogen balance. There really is no downside to the approach. Taking in a little extra protein won't hurt but not getting enough surely will. And in case you're wondering, there is no truth to the claims that higher protein intakes are harmful to the kidneys or bones in healthy people (13), so cross that issue off your worry list.

I've heard some fitness pros claim that a significantly greater protein intake—as much as 2 grams per pound (4.4 g/kg) of body weight—is required to maximize muscle gains. This recommendation conceivably may have credence for those who take performance-enhancing drugs (although such evidence remains purely anecdotal); however, it's excessive if you're not chemically enhanced. The body has a limited capacity to utilize protein for tissue-building purposes, and there's no way to store it for future use. Once this saturation point is reached, additional protein is of no use to your muscles and is either oxidized for energy or converted into glucose or fat (although conversion of protein to fat is a difficult process, making this outcome unlikely). Long-term research studies indicate such extremely high protein intakes do not promote further hypertrophic benefits in natural lifters (1, 2). Moreover, protein tends to blunt appetite, making it difficult for some to take in sufficient calories to support maximal muscle building when protein consumption is excessive.

Much has been made about the importance of consuming high-quality proteins for building muscle. Supplement companies, in particular, have perpetuated the belief that protein quality is paramount, citing qualitative measurement scales such as biological value and protein efficiency ratio to bolster their case. The claims make for good ad copy, but generally speaking the practical implications are wildly overstated.

The quality of a protein is largely a function of its composition of essential amino acids, both in terms of quantity and proportion. A complete protein contains a full complement of all nine essential amino acids in the approximate amounts needed by the body. Conversely, proteins that are low in one or more of the essential amino acids are considered incomplete.

With the exception of gelatin, all animal-based proteins (meats, dairy products, eggs, etc.) are complete proteins. Assuming that you eat a variety of animal-based foods (and follow my recommendation for consuming approximately 1 gram of protein per pound [2.2 g/kg] of body weight), qualitative issues are basically moot; you are assured of getting all the essential amino acids you need for optimal muscle development.

Vegetable-based proteins, on the other hand, tend to lack various essential amino acids; therefore, they are incomplete. This isn't really an issue for lacto-ovo vegetarians because eggs and dairy products contain a full complement of amino acids. Vegans, on the other hand, have to be a little more watchful in regard to protein consumption. They must eat the right combination of foods to ensure they obtain adequate essential amino acids through their diet. For instance, grains are limited in lysine and threonine, whereas legumes are low in methionine. Combining the two offsets the limitations of each and thereby helps prevent a deficiency. Note that these foods don't necessarily have to be eaten in the same meal; they just need to be included in the diet on a regular basis.

CARBOHYDRATE

The recent low-carbohydrate craze has perpetuated the belief that carbohydrate is responsible for pretty much every dietary-related health issue known to humankind. This premise has spawned an entire industry of best-selling books and low-carbohydrate supplements that further the anti-carbohydrate sentiment. As a result, carbophobia runs rampant in a segment of the population. This is especially true for bodybuilders and other physique athletes, who often hold fast to the belief that reducing carbohydrate intake is the key to staying lean.

Let's be clear: Losing body fat is far more complex than simply eliminating carbohydrate from your diet (revisit the first law of thermodynamics, discussed in this chapter). Carbohydrate, when eaten sensibly, can (and likely should) be an integral part of your dietary regimen. This appears particularly true when your goal is to build muscle. To understand why, it's necessary to delve into a little nutritional physiology.

The compounds derived from carbohydrate breakdown are stored as glycogen in your muscles and liver. Glycogen is the primary fuel used to power your muscles during resistance training workouts. It provides an instant source of energy that can be accessed on demand, enabling you to work out at an intense level. As much as 80 percent of the energy used during bodybuilding-style training is derived from muscle glycogen stores (29). Accordingly, multiple research studies show impaired effects on anaerobic performance when a person trains in a glycogen-depleted state (21, 30, 33). Low glycogen levels can be particularly detrimental when you are performing higher-volume routines because the reduced energy availability hastens the onset of fatigue, potentially blunting gains (55, 62).

That said, you don't need to consume a boatload of carbs to achieve optimal performance-related benefits. For example, a diet consisting of 65 percent carbohydrate was shown to have no greater effect on the amount of work performed during 15 sets of 15RM lower-body exercise compared to consuming 40 percent carbohydrate (38). Similarly, physically active men following a moderate-carb diet (50 percent of total calories) performed comparably to when on a high-carb diet (70 percent of total calories) during a bout of supramaximal exercise; alternatively, a low-carb diet consisting of 25 percent of total calories significantly impaired performance (34).

A fairly wide range of carbohydrate intakes can be employed for muscle-building purposes; as with most aspects of nutrition, there are interindividual differences in response to consumption, and you have to figure out what works best for your own body. In my experience, most people seem to do best consuming 2-3 grams of carbohydrate per pound of body weight (4.4-6.6 g/kg). Because each gram of carbohydrate contains four calories, this translates to a daily carbohydrate intake of approximately 1,600-2,400 calories for someone weighing 200 pounds. Those who are insulin insensitive (characterized by an impaired ability to store carbohydrate in the muscles) may require a somewhat lower intake to avoid excess fat storage—perhaps as low as 1 gram per pound (2.2 g/kg) of body weight per day. Experiment with different amounts and see what works best for you.

All types of carbohydrate, however, are not created equal. Some are superior to others for maximizing muscle development while minimizing fat deposition. The best way to determine which types to eat and which to avoid is to assess their nutrient density, a metric that takes into account the number of micronutrients (vitamins, minerals, fiber, etc.) in a food source when considered as a proportion of its caloric content. Nutrient-dense carbohydrates supply your body with essential compounds that enhance metabolic function. Many of the vitamins and minerals in these foods are used as cofactors that assist the body in burning fat. Others act as antioxidants to keep cells functioning optimally. Fiber promotes satiety, decreasing the urge to pig out on junk food; it also supports gut health, which has been linked to enhanced physical performance (39). In sum, these nutrients act symbiotically to keep your body operating at peak efficiency, which ultimately facilitates your ability to build muscle.

Alternatively, keep consumption of highly processed foods to a minimum. Such foods are energy dense and nutrient poor, contributing little to biological function—the essence of an "empty calorie." Moreover, extensive processing tends to make foods highly palatable; so much so that they can short-circuit the brain's ability to regulate appetite. The upshot is that, unless you monitor intake carefully, you'll tend to overeat these foods and inevitably pack on unwanted pounds. This phenomenon was elegantly demonstrated in a study from the lab of Kevin Hall, who confined 20 young weight-stable men and women to a metabolic ward and provided them unlimited access to meals containing ultraprocessed and unprocessed foods in a crossover fashion (19). The meals were equated for calories, sugar, fat, fiber, and macronutrients, but they could eat as many meals as they desired, thus helping to ensure that any observed differences in results could be attributed to the amount eaten of the ultraprocessed versus unprocessed foods. After 14 days, the ultraprocessed meals resulted in an excess intake of approximately 500 calories per day. Moreover, the extra calories correlated with changes in body weight; the ultraprocessed meals brought about a weight gain of nearly 2 pounds (0.9 kg) while the meals of unprocessed foods caused a loss of about the same amount.

Bottom line: Food quality matters!

To ensure your diet is nutrient dense, focus on eating mostly whole or minimally processed foods. Whole grains, fruits, and vegetables should be staple carbohydrates in a muscle-building diet. With respect to packaged foods, learn to read labels. As a general rule, the fewer ingredients in a food source, the less processed it usually is.

That said, you don't necessarily have to cut out all treats. I subscribe to the 80/20 principle; consume 80 percent of your diet from minimally processed foods and then feel free to eat whatever you like for the remaining 20 percent. Consuming the occasional slice of pizza or pint of ice cream won't have any negative effects on your physique, provided you stay within your target caloric intake over time. In fact, satisfying your cravings can actually have a positive effect on your mindset about eating and hence help to maintain long-term dietary adherence.

FAT

Just as some people consider carbohydrate the root of all nutritional evil, others espouse that dietary fat is the biggest culprit in obesity and disease. The low-fat dietary philosophy is predicated on the fact that dietary fat is calorically dense: Each gram contains nine calories. Do the math and you'll see that you have to eat more than twice the amount of protein or carbohydrate (which both have only four calories per gram) to get the same number of calories as a given portion of fat. What's more, consumption of excess fat calories has an almost perfect conversion efficiency, whereas the overconsumption of carbs is met with greater carbohydrate oxidation (31), meaning that it's easier for the body to convert dietary fat into flab than to convert carbohydrate into flab. These factors seem to suggest that a low-fat approach is the key to staying lean.

Unfortunately, these numbers don't tell the whole story and must be considered in the context of a muscle-building diet. Fats are essential nutrients that play a vital role in many body functions. They are involved in cushioning and protecting your internal organs, aiding in the absorption of vitamins, and facilitating the production of cell membranes, hormones, and prostaglandins. Depending on the extent of restriction, low-fat diets can fail to supply the necessary nutrients to keep your body running at peak efficiency and ultimately cause health-related issues.

Low-fat diets may be particularly detrimental to gaining lean mass. Fat consumption is positively associated with testosterone production; if fat intake is restricted, testosterone levels decline. Research shows that the correlation between testosterone levels and fat intake appears to be especially strong in experienced lifters (51). The thing is, despite a lowering of total testosterone, the average values in this research remained well within a normal physiological range (about 300-800 ng/dl for men). While there is no doubt that chronic testosterone levels play a role in muscle development, it's less clear the extent to which fluctuations of the hormone within its normal physiological range has an appreciable impact on gains. Regardless, it's better to err on the side of caution because there's a potential upside to maintaining higher testosterone concentrations without any downside.

Alternatively, diets very high in fat have been shown to actually suppress testosterone levels (61). There appears to be an upper and lower threshold for dietary fat intake to optimize testosterone production, above or below which hormone production may be impaired (51). Taking all factors into account, a moderate approach to fat consumption is therefore warranted. A good rule of thumb is to consume at least 20 percent of calories from fat. Given that mass-building diets require a surplus of calories, this should be fairly easy to accomplish.

Because protein intake is always a constant (approximately 1 g/lb of body weight), the actual number of fat grams consumed is inversely correlated with carbohydrate intake: Consume more carbohydrate and you'll necessarily consume less dietary fat, and vice versa. To determine actual intake, figure out your protein and carbohydrate consumption; your fat consumption will be whatever is left over within your total daily caloric needs. Say, for example, that you weigh 200 pounds (91 kg), and your target is 4,000 calories per day. If you consume 2 grams of carbohydrate per pound of body weight at four calories per gram (1,600 calories) and 1 gram of protein per pound of body weight at four calories per gram (800 calories), then daily fat intake would equal 1,600 calories. Because fat has nine calories per gram, this would equal approximately 178 grams of fat. If you increase carbohydrate intake to 3 grams per pound of body weight, then you reduce fat intake to 800 calories (approximately 89 grams of fat).

The majority of your fats should come from unsaturated sources. Unsaturated fats help maintain fluidity in cell membranes, allowing hormones and other chemical messengers to readily penetrate the cells. This has wide-ranging effects, from increasing muscle protein synthesis to improving insulin sensitivity to enhancing fat utilization.

Monounsaturated fats (found in olive oil, avocado, and various nuts) and polyunsaturated fatty acids (including omega-3 fats derived from fatty fish) are particularly beneficial to cellular processes. In addition to their role in anabolic function, these fats possess health-related benefits that affect virtually every organ system in your body. Suffice to say, they should make up the majority of your dietary fat intake.

There is conflicting evidence about the effects of the intake of saturated fat—found primarily in meats and dairy products—on markers of health.

Some studies show a strong link to cardiovascular diseases and certain types of cancers, whereas others do not. Individual genetics may play a role in the process. A complete discussion of the topic is beyond the scope of this book.

Regardless of the health-related implications, saturated fats contribute little to bodily processes. If not used immediately for energy, they're shuttled with a high degree of efficiency into fat cells for long-term storage. Numerous animal studies have demonstrated that given the same caloric intake, eating saturated fats results in a greater body fat deposition than eating unsaturated fats (18, 42, 57). Moreover, evidence shows that a high intake of saturated fat can reduce insulin sensitivity (47).

The type of dietary fat appears to be particularly important in a bulking phase that involves consuming a surplus of calories. To illustrate, a study by Rosqvist and colleagues (49) overfed a group of subjects by enriching muffins with either a polyunsaturated fat (sunflower oil) or a saturated fat (palmitic acid). After seven weeks, both groups gained an average of 2.2 percent body weight. However, the body composition changes were markedly different between conditions. The group consuming the palmitic acid showed a twofold greater increase in abdominal fat compared to those receiving the calories as sunflower oil. Alternatively, increases in lean mass were approximately threefold greater when consuming sunflower oil.

Bottom line: Focus on consuming unsaturated fats and keep saturated fat intake to a minimum.

SUMMARY OF NUTRITIONAL RECOMMENDATIONS

- If you have relatively little lifting experience, aim to consume a surplus of approximately 500-1,000 calories a day; alternatively, if you're an experienced lifter, the daily surplus should be in a range of approximately 250-500 calories. Use the rule of 100 to adjust caloric intake based on your progress over time.

- Consume approximately 1 gram of protein per pound of body weight.

- Consume approximately 2-3 grams of carbohydrate per pound of body weight. The majority of carbs should come from nutrient-dense sources, including whole grains, fruits, and vegetables.

- After you determine carbohydrate and protein intake, fat intake will constitute the remaining calories in your diet. A minimum intake of approximately 20 percent of total calories is recommended. The majority of fats should come from unsaturated sources, particularly monounsaturated fats and omega-3 fats; minimize intake of saturated fats.

OTHER NUTRITIONAL CONSIDERATIONS

Although energy and macronutrient intake are unquestionably the most important dietary concerns from a hypertrophy standpoint, factors related to temporal aspects of food consumption also can play a role in the process. What follows is a discussion of how these factors can influence muscle building, with evidence-based guidelines provided for optimizing results.

MEAL FREQUENCY

We've covered the basics of what you should eat to pack on mass. Now let's delve into the nuances of how to structure your meals over the course of a day for maximal hypertrophic effect.

Although numerous studies have been carried out to determine the effects of meal frequency on fat loss, there's a dearth of research investigating the topic in regard to gaining muscle while in an energy surplus. Thus, in the absence of controlled evidence, we must defer to logical reasoning to draw conclusions and formulate a strategy. Given that the anabolic effect of a protein-rich meal lasts approximately five to six hours (32), it makes sense to eat at least every five hours or so to ensure you remain in a perpetual muscle-building state. Factoring in time to sleep, this equates to consuming at least three meals per day.

Okay, that's a minimum guideline. The question is, could eating more frequent meals produce better results?

Answer: It might.

One relevant issue to take into account is the need to apportion daily protein intake to maximize its anabolic effects. Although claims that only small doses of protein can be absorbed in a meal have been widely overstated (see the sidebar Maximal Protein "Absorption" per Meal in this chapter), there nevertheless is an upper threshold for intake beyond which the amino acids will be oxidized for fuel rather than utilized for muscle-building purposes. If you recall, the recommended daily protein consumption should be about 1 gram per pound of body weight (2.2 g/kg) per day. Thus, a good rule of thumb for maximizing muscle growth is to consume at least four daily meals throughout the day that contain approximately 0.2-0.25 gram per pound (approximately 0.4-0.55 g/kg) of body weight of a high-quality protein source per meal (54). This will supply the body with amino acids in a manner that should maximize their use for lean tissue synthesis while minimizing their oxidation.

Some lifters may indeed benefit from more frequent meals when bulking. Fact is, it can be difficult to ingest the extra calories required to meet mass-building needs, particularly when eating in a somewhat higher energy surplus. This comes down to individual choice and response; there is no evidence that more frequent meals provide any anabolic benefit. If you do opt to consume meals more frequently, simply allocate the total daily protein requirements into proportionally smaller doses to meet your target intake.

MAXIMAL PROTEIN "ABSORPTION" PER MEAL

A common question relates to the quantity of protein that can be used for muscle building from one meal. A popular claim among fitness circles is that your body can only absorb a relatively small amount of protein in a single feeding. The exact dosage varies depending on who's making the claim, but the upper threshold is generally alleged to be somewhere around 20-30 grams of protein per meal.

Reality check: While the claim is widely accepted as fact, it's at best an overextrapolation of findings from the current literature and lacks a practical basis.

First and foremost, note that the term **absorption** refers to the passage of nutrients from the gut into the bloodstream—and in this context, there is virtually no limit to how much protein you can absorb. The only potential issue from an absorption standpoint is if you supplement with individual free-form amino acids. In such a case, the overabundance of the supplemented amino acids in the gut can cause competition at the intestinal wall, causing them to be preferentially absorbed at the expense of other essential amino acids (17). Otherwise, absorption of whole proteins is a moot concern.

The more relevant question here is whether there's an upper limit to how much protein your body can utilize for muscle-building purposes. This question is a lot more complex and, surprisingly, scientific evidence on the topic is rather limited.

Research indicates that consuming four 20-gram servings of whey protein, one serving every three hours after leg extension exercise, results in greater muscle protein synthesis than two 40-gram servings, consumed six hours apart (5). This finding seems to suggest there's no added anabolic benefit to consuming the higher dosage (40 grams) and that the additional amino acids are simply oxidized for energy. Alternatively, other research shows higher levels of muscle protein synthesis when consuming 40 versus 20 grams of whey following performance of a total-body lifting bout (36). It can be speculated that the greater amount of muscle mass activated in the total-body routine allows for greater utilization of amino acids from the ingested protein compared to performing only leg extension exercise.

One of the primary issues in these studies is that the "meals" provided to subjects consisted of only whey protein. Whey is a fast-acting protein that is absorbed at a rate of about 10 grams per hour (8). Thus, a 20-gram whey bolus would be completely absorbed in a two-hour period. Although this rapid assimilation can transiently elevate rates of muscle protein synthesis, it also causes a greater oxidation of the constituent amino acids at higher protein doses and thus may result in a lower net accretion of muscle tissue compared to a slow-absorbing protein source.

Importantly, most real-life meals generally include a variety of whole foods containing both carbs and fats along with the protein component. This combination of nutrients substantially slows down digestion. The upshot is a more time-released absorption of amino acids into the body, potentially allowing for a greater per-meal dosage without undue amino acid oxidation. This hypothesis is supported by findings of a study comparing consumption of 40 versus 70 grams of protein after performance of a total-body resistance training bout (27). Protein provision was in

(continued)

Maximal Protein "Absorption" per Meal *(continued)*

the form of beef patties consumed with a mixed meal that contained ample amounts of carbs and fat. Results showed that while both protein doses elicited increases in whole-body nitrogen balance, the higher dosage promoted a significantly greater anabolic response, largely attributed to a greater reduction in protein breakdown.

Considering the limitations of the body of literature, here's the take-home message: While certainly a threshold exists beyond which protein will be oxidized for energy rather than used for tissue-building purposes, the amount appears to be well above the often-cited limit of 20-30 grams—with the caveat that nutrients are obtained from whole food–based mixed meals (54). Several variables ultimately influence the metabolism of protein, including the source of protein, the composition of the meal, the dose of the protein or amino acids consumed, and the amount of muscle mass worked in a preceding exercise session. Moreover, individual factors such as age, training status, and the amount of lean body mass also come into play. Thus, the actual limit to how much protein can be utilized will vary somewhat from person to person.

INTERMITTENT FASTING

You might be wondering whether intermittent fasting (a.k.a. time-restricted feeding) might be a viable approach for bulking. In simple terms, intermittent fasting involves limiting food intake to a fairly narrow daily window (usually between four to eight hours) and then abstaining from food the rest of the day. It's a popular strategy for weight loss, and some find it beneficial to help in controlling caloric consumption.

Several studies have been carried out to determine the effects of intermittent fasting on lean mass gains. Early research showed a four-hour time-restricted feeding window was suboptimal in this regard when compared to a traditional meal frequency (59). Alternatively, studies investigating a restricted feeding window of eight hours do not seem to show detrimental effects on lean mass (40, 60). However, note that these studies were not bulking interventions per se; they simply sought to compare body composition changes between intermittent fasting protocols and traditional eating strategies. Given that the studies observed reductions in body fat, it can be inferred that a majority of subjects were in fact in a caloric deficit during the intervention period. Thus, relevant conclusions cannot be drawn about maximizing hypertrophy.

From a practical standpoint, it's difficult to take in sufficient calories over short time periods; this tends to make intermittent fasting unfeasible for bulking purposes. Moreover, there appears to be a benefit to spreading out protein intake evenly across the day as opposed to concentrating consumption in a limited time frame (63). Thus, while intermittent fasting may help some people limit food intake when attempting to lose body fat, it's generally not an ideal approach if your goal is to maximize muscular gains.

NUTRIENT TIMING AND THE ANABOLIC BARN DOOR THEORY

For many years, the concept of an "anabolic window of opportunity" was accepted as gospel in the fitness field. Simply stated, the theory espouses that the body is in a hyper-anabolic state immediately following the performance of exercise. According to its proponents, protein and carbs therefore must be consumed within 45-60 minutes post-workout to maximize exercise-induced adaptations; delay consumption of nutrients beyond this narrow window and you'll go catabolic, sacrificing potential muscular gains.

When writing the first edition of this book (circa 2010), I bought into the anabolic window theory hook, line, and sinker. As such, I harped on the importance of ingesting nutrients as quickly as possible after a workout. The recommendation seemed like a no-brainer. I'd seen a number of studies suggesting the presence of a narrow post-exercise window. I'd read the seminal text, *Nutrient Timing: The Future of Sports Nutrition*, by John Ivy and Robert Portman that extolled the approach (23). I'd heard a number of prominent researchers in the field champion the theory at conferences. Heck, one of the major sports nutrition organizations devoted an entire position stand to the topic (26). Suffice to say, the supporting evidence seemed pretty overwhelming.

Following publication of this book's first edition, however, I got around to chatting with my colleague, über sports nutritionist Alan Aragon. During the course of our conversation, he questioned the relevance of the anabolic window, pointing to confounding issues and limitations in the interpretation of data. It caught me off guard at first; could it be that the consensus of virtually the entire scientific community was off base? As an ever-curious scientist, I was skeptical but open to changing my opinion. The discussion spurred me to revisit the topic. I delved into the literature, poring over every relevant study I could find.

Lo and behold, the more I read, the less convinced I became of the veracity of the supporting evidence.

Clearly, there was compelling research showing that resistance exercise sensitizes muscle to the anabolic effects of food; however, this sensitization lasts at least 24 hours post-workout (10). It became increasingly evident that the anabolic window theory was largely based on results from acute studies (research investigating the effects of timing after a single exercise bout). These types of studies use surrogate markers of hypertrophy (such as intracellular signaling or muscle protein synthesis) to draw conclusions about muscular adaptations. The problem is, while such studies are beneficial for drawing hypotheses, their findings cannot necessarily be extrapolated to long-term results. The only way to determine causality on the topic is with longitudinal studies that actually measure changes in muscle growth over time. And in this regard, one thing that really struck me was the disparity in findings from longitudinal studies; some showed a hypertrophic benefit to immediate post-exercise protein provision while others did not.

In an effort to provide clarity as to the validity of a narrow window of opportunity for anabolism, our group carried out a meta-analysis where we pooled data from all studies on the topic (52). We considered only studies that compared rapid intake of protein pre- or post-exercise (≤1 hour) versus delaying consumption (>2 hours); a total of 23 trials met inclusion criteria encompassing over 500 participants. Interestingly, the initial basic analysis did in fact show a small but statistically significant effect on muscle hypertrophy. Had we effectively confirmed the existence of an anabolic window?

As it turned out, that conclusion proved premature.

We next performed a regression analysis whereby a number of variables (i.e., covariates) were examined independently to evaluate their impact on results. This produced the most interesting finding of all: The total daily protein intake of subjects explained virtually all the variance in results! Specifically, a majority of studies did not match protein intake between groups: The protein timing group consumed substantially more protein than the controls (1.7 g/kg/day versus 1.3 g/kg/day, respectively). Thus, the average protein consumption in the control groups was well below that deemed necessary to maximize training-induced muscle protein synthesis. Only a few studies actually endeavored to match intake. We carried out a subanalysis of these studies; no effects were found from protein timing.

Now the findings of our meta-analysis come with an important caveat. Namely, our criterion for timed consumption was ≤1 hour pre- or post-workout, while the nontimed groups was >2 hours. We therefore were not able to determine if waiting, say, five hours or more to eat after a training session would have a negative impact. Based on the literature, we'd previously proposed that a window probably exists, but it is rather wide (four to six hours) and ultimately depends on when you ate your pre-workout meal (4). That hypothesis remained to be tested.

So, we subsequently set out to conduct a study to determine if in fact the timing of the pre-workout meal influenced the need to consume protein quickly post-exercise (53). The study randomized resistance-trained men to receive a supplement containing 25 grams of whey protein either immediately before or immediately after an intense workout. Participants receiving the supplement prior to training were instructed to refrain from eating for at least three hours after their sessions to ensure post-exercise nutrition did not confound results. Similarly, those receiving the supplement after training were instructed to refrain from eating for at least three hours prior to the sessions to avoid confounding results from pre-exercise nutrition. At the end of the 10-week study period, increases in muscle mass were similar between groups, indicating that any benefits of immediate post-workout protein consumption are negated when you take in sufficient protein prior to training.

The overall take-home message from the scientific literature is that there isn't a narrow anabolic window of opportunity; for the vast majority of the population, it really doesn't matter whether you consume protein immediately after training or delay consumption for a few hours. This should be liberating for most lifters. You don't have to stress about slamming a shake the minute you finish lifting. It's okay to relax a bit, do whatever you need to do, and get in your post-workout nutrition when it's most convenient. Much more important is to make sure you meet your minimum daily protein requirements as previously discussed.

With that said, it makes sense to err on the side of caution and consume protein relatively quickly after training, provided your goal is to maximize muscle growth—and if you're reading this book, I'd assume that's the case. Although the findings of our meta-analysis did not show statistical differences between timing versus untimed strategies, we couldn't rule out that a slight benefit may in fact exist to early post-exercise protein provision. There is a potential upside and really no downside, making for a good cost–benefit ratio. So, while you don't need to freak out if you're not able to take in protein immediately post-workout, it's better not to wait too long. Certainly, delaying nutrient consumption for many hours after training is unwise.

Okay, so we can safely say that the importance of consuming protein immediately post-exercise has been overstated. But what about carbohydrate intake? The anabolic window theory posits that ingesting carbs with protein in the post-exercise period produces a synergistic hypertrophic response. This is largely based on the premise that carbohydrate stimulates insulin, which has known anticatabolic properties that help to attenuate muscle protein breakdown following a workout (9).

Although the theory has a sound logical rationale, there's an important issue that's often overlooked: Protein also is a potent stimulator of insulin. In fact, a 45-gram dose of whey protein produces a rise in levels sufficient to maximize the anticatabolic response to training (45). As you therefore might expect, both acute (16, 20, 28, 56) and long-term (22) studies have failed to show an additive anabolic benefit of combined post-exercise protein and carb consumption versus consuming protein alone.

Another proposed reason for consuming carbs immediately after training is to replete glycogen stores. As previously mentioned, bodybuilding-type training is largely fueled by muscle glycogen. Substantial depletion of glycogen stores occurs after an intense training session, particularly when performing relatively high training volumes (48). Indeed, research indicates a supercompensation of muscle glycogen stores when carbs are ingested immediately after exercise; delaying intake by just two hours diminishes the rate of resynthesis by approximately 50 percent (24). Moreover, consuming a combination of protein and carbs post-workout enhances the rate of resynthesis over and above consuming carbohydrate alone (7).

Given the importance of glycogen to resistance training performance, this may seem like a big deal. However, the need for rapid repletion of glycogen stores generally has little relevance if your goal is to maximize muscle growth.

Here's the rub.

Assuming total carbohydrate intake is equal across the course of a day, glycogen repletion is similar after 24 hours regardless of whether carbs are consumed immediately after training or if intake is delayed by several hours (43). Even if your glycogen stores are fully depleted—which is highly doubtful in traditional resistance training routines—restoration occurs well within this time frame, irrespective of the timing of carb intake after exercise (14). Thus, unless you're performing two-a-day splits for the same muscle group(s), it really doesn't matter much how quickly you take in carbs after a workout provided total daily intake needs are met.

In sum, emerging evidence over the past decade indicates a new paradigm in nutrient timing theory: The anabolic "window" of opportunity is really more of an anabolic "barn door." Ultimately, the need to take in nutrients quickly after a workout will depend on when you consume a pre-workout meal. Accordingly, think of your meals as brackets around training sessions. You remain in an anabolic state for approximately 5-6 hours following a protein-rich meal, with the duration dependent on the composition of the meal (i.e., total amount of protein, nutrient quality, energy content, etc.). Thus, if you eat breakfast at, say, seven a.m., then train for an hour at nine a.m., you conceivably have at least several hours to consume a post-exercise meal without compromising gains. Provided you follow the general nutrition recommendations laid out in this book and train between breakfast and dinner, you'll necessarily be within your anabolic window. Alternatively, if you train first thing in the morning before breakfast, then there's a heightened benefit to consuming protein relatively quickly post-workout.

TAKE-HOME POINTS ABOUT NUTRIENT TIMING

■ Aim to consume at least four daily meals with the protein content spread out fairly evenly across the day.

■ Nutrient timing can be a beneficial strategy for maximizing muscular gains, but the "window" of opportunity is really more of a "barn door," where muscle tissue is sensitized to nutrient intake for several hours post-workout.

■ Provided that a protein-rich meal is consumed within about three to four hours prior to a workout (or possibly even longer, depending on the size of the meal), you don't have to stress about chowing down a post-workout meal as soon as you finish training. For those who train partially or fully fasted, on the other hand, consuming protein immediately post-workout becomes increasingly more important to promote anabolism.

■ If your goal is to maximize muscle development, it seems prudent to consume high-quality protein (at a dose of approximately 0.2-0.25 g/lb [approximately 0.4-0.5 g/kg] of lean body mass) relatively quickly after a workout. Although evidence is somewhat equivocal, there is a potential (albeit small) benefit to the approach without any downside.

■ Contrary to popular belief, consuming post-exercise carbohydrate does not meaningfully enhance anabolism. Moreover, unless you are performing two workouts a day involving the same muscle group(s), glycogen replenishment will not be a limiting factor provided you consume sufficient carbohydrate over the course of a given day. So, from a muscle-building standpoint, just focus on meeting your daily carb requirement as opposed to worrying about timing issues.

THE CARDIO CONNECTION

By this point you've learned how the M.A.X. Muscle Plan's systematically structured combination of periodized resistance training and proper nutrition helps maximize muscle development. If you follow the program as directed, you're bound to see terrific results.

But what about cardio or, more precisely, exercise that stresses the heart and lungs? Can adding some aerobic exercise to the mix be of further benefit? The answer is a qualified "yes," provided you adhere to some basic guidelines.

PROS AND CONS OF CARDIO FOR OPTIMIZING BODY COMPOSITION

Without question, cardiovascular exercise promotes a plethora of health-related benefits, helping to improve both the quality and length of life. That's a given. I'd note, though, that to varying degrees, regular resistance training confers most of these same benefits and more. The benefits of resistance training are multisystemic and multidimensional, extending to virtually every organ system (13); arguably, no other exercise modality has a greater positive impact on overall wellness. That said, including both resistance training and cardio in a structured exercise program promotes synergistic health-related effects that may combine to further reduce the risk of disease. The specifics and nuances of the topic are beyond the scope of this book.

When evaluating the relevance of cardiovascular exercise from a hypertrophy standpoint, we must consider the principle of specificity. If you recall, the principle of specificity states that adaptations are specific to the type of training you perform. With respect to cardio, several associated adaptations can have a beneficial effect on body composition. For one, cardio helps expand your network of capillaries (2)—the tiny blood vessels that allow nutrient exchange between body tissues. Although resistance training alone does promote capillarization, the extent of these increases is limited; only by adding cardio to the mix can you optimally enhance angiogenic adaptations (18).

Capillary increases have particular relevance to fat loss. You see, before body fat can be metabolized, it must first enter the bloodstream and then be transported to the active tissues for use as fuel. Unfortunately, blood flow tends to be poor in fatty areas, which inhibits your body's ability to harness fat from these regions. The more capillaries you have, the more efficient your body becomes at liberating and using fat, particularly from stubborn areas. To this point, fat loss from cardio exercise seems to preferentially come from the midsection, irrespective of dietary factors. Tightly controlled studies on rodents show that performing regular aerobic exercise significantly reduces abdominal fat even when energy intake is kept constant (12). Studies on humans seem to support this finding as well (11), raising the possibility that performing some cardio may help to minimize abdominal fat accretion during a bulking phase.

Moreover, regular aerobic exercise expands the size and number of your mitochondria (cellular furnaces where fat burning takes place) and increases the quantity of your aerobic enzymes (body proteins that accelerate the fat-burning process). It also has a sensitizing effect on insulin function, facilitating the storage of carbohydrate as glycogen rather than as fat. Over time, these factors further ratchet up your body's fat-burning capacity and enhance the potential for recomposition. Intriguingly, mitochondrial dysfunction is associated with increased activation of the intracellular signaling enzyme AMPK (8), which as previously discussed has a catabolic effect on muscle tissue. Thus, by improving mitochondrial function, aerobic training also may indirectly help to enhance anabolic processes and spur muscle growth.

In addition to the aforementioned benefits, cardio aids in recuperation from intense training. The increased blood flow to muscles in combination with greater capillarization enhances delivery of oxygen, growth factors, and macronutrients to damaged fibers, facilitating their ability to remodel. The upshot is faster recovery and hence a better ability to sustain performance over time.

Further, cardio serves as a form of active recovery. During aerobic training, blood is shunted to the working muscles. This further enhances nutrient delivery and facilitates the removal of metabolic by-products; it's why muscle soreness tends to dissipate more quickly after performing a bout of light cardio. The catch is that responses are muscle specific. If you perform only lower-body cardio, you'll see the majority of recovery-related benefits in your legs. To realize results in the upper body, you need to perform upper-body cardio exercises. This generally shouldn't be an issue because many cardio machines, such as elliptical trainers and Arc Trainers, include upper-body components so that all the major muscles are engaged during a workout. No cardio equipment? No problem. Simply pumping your arms while walking achieves similar beneficial effects.

With all these benefits, it seems like adding a cardio component to the M.A.X. Muscle Plan would be a no-brainer, right? Unfortunately, it's not that simple. Concurrently performing aerobic and resistance exercise can in fact compromise muscle growth. This has been dubbed the chronic interference hypothesis, which proposes that trained muscle cannot adapt optimally to the combination of both types of training (19). Depending on the specific training regimen, the negative effect on muscle development can be significant.

The problem with concurrent training is that adaptations associated with resistance training aren't necessarily compatible with those of aerobic exercise. Each type of training regimen activates and suppresses specific genes and signaling pathways, and these pathways tend to interfere with one another. The net result is an impaired adaptive response, particularly from a muscle hypertrophy standpoint; cardio seems to impair resistance training adaptations more than vice versa.

AMPK is generally considered a primary culprit in the interference phenomenon. If you recall, AMPK is associated with an energy-conserving pathway that regulates adenosine triphosphate (ATP), the high-energy compound that fuels all human work. When energy levels become depleted during aerobic exercise, AMPK turns on enzymes involved in carbohydrate and fatty acid metabolism to restore ATP levels. Among other things, this increases the use of fat as a fuel source.

That's the good news.

The bad news is that AMPK activation also blocks an anabolic signaling enzyme called mammalian target of rapamycin (mTOR), which is critical for carrying out muscle protein synthesis. This makes biological sense because the body uses a lot of energy to make muscle proteins, and conserving energy becomes essential to survival during times when ATP levels are low. The interference effects of AMPK on anabolic processes were demonstrated in an elegant study whereby researchers electrically stimulated the hind limb muscles of rats with either long-duration, low frequencies (to simulate aerobic exercise) or short-duration, high frequencies (to simulate resistance training) (1). Results showed that low-frequency stimulation ramped up AMPK whereas high-frequency stimulation activated PKB, an anabolic signaling enzyme. The researchers thus termed the phenomenon the AMPK-PKB switch, which proposes that aerobic and anaerobic exercise produce opposing signaling responses that are incompatible for optimizing muscular adaptations. Now, in reality, the concept of a "switch" that regulates anabolism and catabolism is overly simplistic; considerable overlap exists between strength- and endurance-related responses to exercise. But on a general level the point is clear: Aerobic exercise can interfere with hypertrophic adaptations from resistance training.

Another potential downside to concurrent training is the overtraining factor. Remember that everyone has an upper limit to how much exercise they can tolerate before overtraining sets in. Performing cardio adds to the total amount of exercise-related stress placed on your body. These stresses can overwhelm your capacity to recover, ultimately leading to an overtrained state. Overtraining is associated with heightened fatigue, reduced testosterone levels, increased cortisol levels (a catabolic stress hormone), and an impaired immune response. To say the least, these factors are not conducive to gaining muscle.

All things considered, the addition of cardio can be beneficial to a hyper-trophy-oriented training program. However, to achieve a favorable cost–ben-efit ratio, you must properly manage aerobic training variables in a manner that promotes positive adaptations while minimizing potential interference effects. This requires both insight and planning.

INTEGRATING CARDIO INTO THE M.A.X. MUSCLE PLAN

Assuming you decide to include a cardio component, the routine must be carefully structured to complement the resistance-training element of the M.A.X. Muscle Plan. Cardio has three distinct variables: intensity, volume (combination of duration and frequency), and mode. Intensity and volume will be discussed in the ensuing paragraphs because their manipulation is interrelated; mode will be discussed in a separate section later in the chapter.

1. **Intensity** refers to how hard you train. You can estimate aerobic training intensity in several ways. The most popular method involves taking a per-centage of maximal heart rate (MHR), which is calculated by subtracting your age from 220. For example, if you are 30 years old, your maximal heart rate is 190 (220 – 30 = 190). To determine training intensity, simply multiply this number by a given percentage based on how hard you want to exercise. So let's say you want to perform steady-state cardio at 60 percent max heart rate (a relatively low intensity). Using the previously calculated max heart rate of 190 as an example, your target heart rate would be 114 beats per minute. It's that easy. I'll note that the formula is a bit of an oversimplification because the relationship between max heart rate and age is not necessarily linear and appears to be influenced by fitness level. More detail is beyond the scope of this book, and the stated max heart rate formula is sufficient for our purposes.

   As an alternative to the heart rate method, you can use a rating of perceived exertion (RPE) to gauge aerobic intensity, as described in chapter 6. Simply stated, RPE is a measure of how hard you feel you are exercising. With respect to cardio, RPE takes into account the physical sensations you experience during exercise, including increases in heart rate, breathing rate, sweating, and muscle fatigue. Revisit table 6.1 for specific guidelines on how to estimate RPE when performing cardio. Personally, I prefer the RPE method to max heart rate because it's a more comprehensive measure of the factors involved in intensity. That said, whether you choose to measure intensity by the heart rate or RPE method is completely up to you; both are viable options.

   Aerobic intensity exists on a continuum, with slow walking at one end of the spectrum and an all-out sprint at the opposite end. A strategy called high-intensity interval training (HIIT) incorporates a combination of intensities whereby relatively short bursts of high-intensity aerobic activity are interspersed with periods of low-intensity activity. Examples include alternating periods of running and walking or sprint cycling and easy pedaling; however, any cardio modality can be employed provided it allows the ability to train at varying aerobic intensities.

If you're new to resistance training, adding a cardio component can actually enhance muscle growth; the caveat is that aerobic intensity must be relatively high to achieve results. HIIT has proven particularly effective in this regard (5). Consistent with its endurance-oriented nature, hypertrophy from aerobic training is generally specific to type 1 muscle fibers; type 2 growth is limited (9). Moreover, hypertrophic effects dissipate after a few months because it becomes impossible to progressively overload the muscles in a manner that promotes ongoing adaptations. Thus, your choice of aerobic intensity should not be based on its direct muscle-building effects but rather on the indirect benefits discussed previously. In this regard, similar benefits can be attained across the spectrum of intensity options; let personal preference guide your decision-making.

2. **Volume** of aerobic exercise should be considered on a weekly basis. In this regard, volume represents a combination of aerobic duration and frequency. **Duration** refers to how long you train. As a general rule, duration is inversely related to intensity; you can go longer if you don't train as hard. **Frequency** refers to how often you train. Frequency is generally expressed in terms of the number of weekly aerobic sessions (although technically you could perform multiple sessions in the same day). Thus, volume is calculated as the product of duration and frequency.

Volume may have the greatest influence on the hypertrophic interference associated with concurrent training. When combined with intense lifting sessions, long, frequent aerobic bouts can give rise to a catabolic hormonal environment and chronic muscle glycogen depletion, hastening the onset of overtraining (14). That said, the impact of aerobic volume on gains will depend somewhat on intensity. Most well-trained lifters can take long, leisurely walks on a daily basis without substantially overtaxing their recovery abilities. Alternatively, frequent marathon-type running sessions clearly can interfere with the anabolic process and impair growth (17).

The key to ensuring that hard-earned muscle is not sacrificed in a concurrent training regimen is to strike a balance between cardio intensity and volume. Doing so helps to minimize the effects of chronic interference on anabolic intracellular signaling and reduce the potential for overtraining. Moderation is paramount.

What constitutes moderation? This will somewhat vary from person to person and depends on such factors as individual recovery ability, phase of the resistance training program, and training experience, among others. A rule of thumb is to keep the duration (and hence volume) of aerobic exercise low when intensity is high and vice versa. Thus, you can perform longer sessions if the extent of your cardio involves walking at a modest pace (although at some point extended walking sessions may ultimately interfere with anabolic processes). Alternatively, the duration of HIIT sessions should be kept relatively short. A general recommendation is to limit HIIT to 20 minutes or so—even less if the sessions involve very high-intensity sprints.

As a guideline, limit aerobic frequency to no more than three to four times per week when the intensity of training is moderate to high; from my experience, higher frequencies tend to cause undue fatigue when combined with intensive resistance training, thus impairing muscular gains. That said, the prescription of aerobic frequency will to some extent be dependent on your daily activity levels. Those who are very sedentary, particularly working desk jobs, may benefit from an extra day or so of cardio. Alternatively, if you're highly active in everyday life, it might be best to perform cardio just a day or two per week to ensure that you avoid the potential for chronic interference.

Note that you can choose to employ a variety of aerobic intensities and, correspondingly, volumes as part of a structured cardio routine. For example, you could go for leisurely hour-long jogs a couple of days a week and then perform a 20-minute HIIT session on an alternate day (or vice versa). Remember, though, tolerance will always be specific to the individual. Given that the goal of this program is to build muscle, it's best to err on the side of caution in the initial stages of the program. Begin by performing less intense and lengthy cardio sessions and then gradually adjust the variables over time based on your response.

The phase of the resistance training program also must be considered with respect to aerobic variables. In this regard, it's generally best to curtail the use of HIIT sessions during higher-volume lifting cycles because the competing high intensities of training increase the potential for overtraining. Opt instead for low-intensity steady-state exercise (e.g., walking), which carries a lower risk of chronic interference (3, 4), and alter the duration and frequency of sessions based on your perceived level of fatigue.

TIMING OF CARDIO

Another important consideration of concurrent training is when to perform the cardio component. You have two basic choices:

1. Schedule cardio on your days off from resistance training
2. Include cardio on your lifting day

Which is best? As a general rule, the further you can distance the aerobic bout from your lifting session, the better. Best results are attained by performing cardio and lifting on separate days (19). This is most feasible during phases of the program when you're lifting three days per week, thus allowing four available days to train aerobically. However, the strategy becomes more problematic when performing higher-resistance training frequencies; depending on how many cardio sessions you choose to do, at some point the numbers just won't add up. Moreover, you might want more off days to spend at your leisure as opposed to exercising all the time; personal preference is a huge consideration that must be taken into account in program design.

If you can't (or don't want to) lift and do cardio on separate days, the next-best option is to split up the two components and perform cardio in the morning and resistance train later in the day (or vice versa). This is of particular consequence if you're doing HIIT because research shows training aerobically at high intensities heightens interference when performed in close proximity to a resistance-training bout (7). Provided you're properly managing aerobic volume and intensity, the order in which you perform the bouts doesn't really matter; allowing several hours of inactivity between sessions affords your body time to recover and replenish its resources. However, when performing cardio in the morning before eating, it's beneficial to take in carbohydrate immediately post-exercise to facilitate glycogen repletion, as discussed in chapter 11. Fatigue shouldn't be an issue as long as your nutritional regimen is sound.

If you're unable or unwilling to split up the workouts and have to perform both cardio and resistance training in the same session, make sure to follow one basic rule: Always lift first. The residual fatigue from aerobic training can reduce the amount of volume performed in a subsequent lifting session (7), sabotaging gains. Even relatively low-intensity cardio can sap vital energy reserves. You lose that extra oomph that you could otherwise draw on to push yourself, ultimately reducing the intensity of your lifts. Research indicates that performing cardio prior to resistance training interferes with anabolic signaling, with negative effects seen regardless of whether the bout involves HIIT or moderate-intensity steady-state aerobic exercise (3, 4).

THE FASTED CARDIO MYTH

A popular fat-loss strategy is to perform aerobic exercise first thing in the morning on an empty stomach. The rationale for the strategy is that a prolonged absence of food reduces circulating blood sugar, causing glycogen (stored carbohydrate) levels to fall. With less available glycogen, your body has no choice but to rely more on fat, rather than glucose, to fuel your workout. Moreover, the low insulin levels associated with fasting promote an environment that is favorable to fat breakdown, increasing the availability of fatty acids to be used as energy during the exercise session.

Unfortunately, what may seem like a sound strategy doesn't seem to transfer into practice. Studies show that although a greater breakdown of fat takes place when you have fasted than after you have eaten, the rate of breakdown exceeds

(continued)

The Fasted Cardio Myth *(continued)*

your body's ability to burn the extra fatty acids for fuel (6, 10). In other words, a lot of extra fatty acids that the working muscles can't use are floating around in the blood. Ultimately, these fatty acids are repackaged into triglycerides during the post-workout period and then shuttled back into fat cells. In the end, you've gone to excessive lengths only to wind up at the same place you started.

More importantly, it's shortsighted to simply look at the number of fat calories you burn during an exercise session. Your metabolism doesn't operate in a vacuum. Rather, the body continually adjusts its use of fat and carbohydrate for fuel depending on a variety of factors. As a general rule, if you burn more carbohydrate during an exercise session, you'll ultimately burn a greater amount of fat in the post-workout period, and vice versa (15). This begs the question, who cares if you burn a few extra fat calories while exercising if the ratio shifts to a greater carbohydrate utilization an hour later? In the end, it doesn't make a bit of difference. Bottom line: You need to evaluate fat burning over the course of days, not on an hour-to-hour basis, to get a meaningful perspective on its effect on body composition.

To determine the efficacy of fasted cardio as a fat-loss strategy, our lab carried out a controlled study that randomized a cohort of young women to perform cardio three days a week in either a fed or fasted state (16). For each workout, both groups came to the lab in the morning without eating. The fed group then received a shake containing carbs and protein prior to performing 60 minutes of moderate-intensity aerobic exercise on a treadmill while the fasted group consumed the same shake after the workout. After four weeks, results showed similar reductions in body fat between groups, indicating no benefit to performing cardio on an empty stomach.

One potential issue sometimes raised is the effect of fasted cardio on muscle proteins. Research indicates that nitrogen losses more than double when performing moderate-intensity cardio when muscle glycogen is depleted compared to glycogen loaded (19). While on the surface these findings seem to suggest a detriment to programs designed to maximize muscle mass, it should be noted that an overnight fast depletes liver glycogen stores but has limited effect on muscle glycogen. Thus, the findings cannot necessarily be interpreted to imply that fasted cardio is catabolic to muscle development.

Bottom line: Although research remains limited on the topic, it seems safe to say that if there are any body composition benefits from fasted cardio (still highly equivocal), they would be minor at best. On the other hand, the strategy doesn't seem to be detrimental. Thus, whether you perform cardio fasted or fed should depend entirely on preference, not on the belief that it will get you shredded.

CHOOSING A CARDIO MODE

Cardio can be carried out using a variety of different modes. The choices include a panoply of different types of aerobic equipment, such as treadmills, stationary cycles, stair climbers, and elliptical trainers. If you prefer outdoor activities, jogging, hiking, and cycling are attractive options. Other aerobic alternatives include skipping or jumping rope and various calisthenic exercises (e.g., jumping jacks). The options are vast and varied.

Generally speaking, you should choose a modality based on preference. The most important factor in getting results is adherence, and if you like the cardio modality, you'll be more inclined to stick with it over time. That said, there are considerations that should be taken into account from a cost–benefit perspective. Most specifically, some research indicates that running may be especially detrimental to muscle growth when performed in combination with resistance exercise (19). It is speculated that running-related impairments to hypertrophy may be related to excessive muscle damage caused by higher associated eccentric forces compared to other modes. Conceivably, high levels of damage could interfere with post-exercise recovery and thus blunt muscular adaptations. Alternatively, cycling appears to interfere less with resistance training–induced hypertrophy. This has been attributed to greater biomechanical similarities between cycling and multi-joint lower-body free weight exercise compared to running, which in turn may promote a better transfer of training (19). However, these conclusions were based on a limited amount of data and thus should be viewed with a degree of circumspection.

Given the relative paucity of evidence on the topic, it's difficult to draw strong conclusions on whether one cardio mode is superior to another in the context of a hypertrophy-oriented concurrent training program. That said, consistent with the adage, "When in doubt, leave it out," it seems prudent to avoid, or at least substantially limit, running or sprinting when the goal is to maximize muscle growth; inclusion of these activities has a potential downside with no logical upside. If you opt to perform HIIT-style cardio, numerous viable alternatives exist to achieve desired results.

CHAPTER 13

THE M.A.X. MUSCLE PLAN 2.0 Q&A

The following are answers to common questions that I've received since publication of the first edition of this book.

Question: *I'm in my fifties. Are there any modifications that I should make to the program?*

Answer: The aging process most certainly takes a toll on the body in a manner that alters its response to exercise training. In simple terms, your hypertrophic potential becomes blunted with advancing age, which is known as age-related "anabolic insensitivity." There are several contributory reasons for this phenomenon. For one, chronic levels of anabolic hormones fall precipitously with age. In men, there is a substantial decline in testosterone that accelerates exponentially in the later stages of life; in postmenopausal women, estrogen levels (the primary female anabolic hormone) are reduced by as much as one-tenth of that before menopause. Moreover, the number of satellite cells decreases with advancing age, particularly in the larger type II muscle fibers, as does their ability to activate and proliferate. The upshot is an impaired capacity for synthesizing muscle proteins. On top of everything, joint-related issues such as osteoarthritis become more prevalent, hindering the ability to train with heavy loads and high levels of effort.

While these issues may seem daunting, take heart that you can continue to build muscle into your golden years. Research shows that even the oldest of old achieve substantial hypertrophy when they adhere to a regimented resistance training program, just to a lesser extent than younger lifters. Still, there are some things to keep in mind as you get older that may require modifying certain aspects of the M.A.X. Muscle Plan.

First, recovery abilities generally diminish with age, and it thus tends to take longer to restore performance to baseline levels. These impairments may be a function of greater muscle damage from training or a heightened fatigue response, or both. Regardless of the mechanism, older individuals therefore need to place a greater focus on managing recovery and may benefit from performing fewer weekly training sessions to allow for regeneration of neuromuscular capacity. It also may be helpful to engage in various post-workout recovery strategies such as hot baths, foam rolling, or massage. The effectiveness of these strategies remains somewhat equivocal, but some claim to achieve positive benefits from their use. There is little downside, so give them a try to see if they are of benefit to you.

Second, you may not be able to tolerate as much volume as when you were younger. Although it's difficult to provide specific guidelines, volume reductions of 25-50 percent are often necessary to avoid nonfunctional overreaching as lifters progress from their 30s and 40s to their 60s and 70s. You need to listen to your body and be in tune with how it responds to the cumulative effects of the program. If you feel the amount of volume is causing undue fatigue, reduce the number of sets accordingly.

Third, it may be advisable to reduce or even eliminate very heavy loads. Most older individuals probably should avoid training at their 1RM during the strength phase and focus on the three to five rep range (although this will be somewhat dependent on the individual). If you have an existing joint-related condition, you may need to skip the strength phase altogether. While this may somewhat negatively impact the potentiation effect on the muscle phase of the program, you're better off erring on the side of caution. Remember, you can't make gains when suffering from a debilitating injury that derails your training efforts.

Finally, the number of so-called "poor responders" to resistance training increases in older individuals. That said, assuming there are no underlying medical conditions, everyone can ultimately build appreciable muscle, regardless of age and genetics. It's just a matter of figuring out how your body responds to stimuli. Thus, you might need to experiment a bit more with manipulating variables to determine what works best for you.

It's important to appreciate the fact that the response to aging varies greatly between individuals. In this regard, you must take into account chronological age (your actual age in years) versus biological age (a function of physical and mental capacity). I've known people in their 70s who have a greater muscle-building capacity and fitness level than some in their 20s. If you've followed a healthy lifestyle over the years, it's likely you have aged better than someone who did not. So while chronological age is a factor that warrants consideration, also consider your biological age from a programming standpoint.

Question: *Are there any differences between men and women that should be considered when performing the program?*

Answer: Relative increases in hypertrophy (on a percentage basis from baseline) are similar between the sexes when following a regimented resistance training program. However, this must be understood in the context that women start off with less muscle mass at baseline, thus biasing percentage increases in their favor. From an absolute standpoint, muscular gains are significantly greater in men than in women, conceivably explained to a large extent by differences in chronic testosterone production (women have about one-tenth the circulating testosterone levels of men). Bottom line: While women can build appreciable muscle, their absolute hypertrophic potential is somewhat less on average than that of men.

For the most part, the approach to training is quite similar between men and women; thus, the program will work equally well, regardless of sex. That said, it's relevant to note that women tend to display faster recovery than men between sets of moderate- to high-rep training. It's believed this may be due, at least in part, to the fact that women generally use lighter weights, which reduces the level of post-set stress to the neuromuscular system. Other factors may also be involved, perhaps related to hormonal differences. Regardless, women therefore may be able to employ somewhat shorter rest intervals in the metabolic and muscle phases without compromising muscle development. At the very least, this allows for a greater training efficiency, reducing the time required to optimize results.

Question: *Is it necessary to do the strength and metabolic phases? Can't I just do the muscle phase?*

Answer: I realize it can be tempting to solely focus on the muscle phase, since the name of the phase implies it's solely responsible for maximizing growth. However, that's not the case. Understand that the phases of the program are designed to interact synergistically, with each phase potentiating the next to enhance the ultimate effects on muscle development. Omitting a phase thus can actually impair your ability to achieve maximal gains.

It's essential to look at muscle building as a process that necessarily involves preparatory work to reach your goal. Although almost everyone is driven to get results as quickly as possible, you must allow the process to run its course; attempting to take shortcuts inevitably shortchanges results. If desired, you may be able to get away with shortening the strength phase to four or six weeks instead of eight without any detriment. This will largely depend on your initial strength levels. Those who possess a high level of strength when beginning the program, particularly those who have regularly engaged in powerlifting or strongman or strongwoman training, generally won't be negatively impacted by reducing the length of the strength phase. Alternatively, if your strength levels are on the low side, you'd likely benefit from going through the entire phase as outlined. Just try to be as objective as possible and avoid allowing impulsiveness to unduly influence decision-making.

Question: *Is it necessary to do maximum lifts in the strength phase? I don't have a spotter and feel uncomfortable performing a 1RM.*

Answer: The closer you train to your 1RM, the greater the transfer of strength to your lifts. This is a basic extrapolation of the principle of specificity. Thus, there's a benefit to at least occasionally performing max lifts during the strength phase; it's consistent with the goal of the phase.

That said, strength is achieved on a continuum whereby the closer you train to your 1RM, the greater the strength transfer. Hence, you will achieve most strength gains from training in a loading zone of three to five reps per set as you would from performing max lifts. If there's a specific reason why you prefer to avoid performing 1RMs (and not having a spotter is a good reason, as are the issues associated with advanced aging mentioned earlier in the Q&A), feel free to stay with the three to five rep range. Although you might compromise strength gains a tad, the overall difference should be of minimal consequence and likely have little to no detrimental impact on potentiating the muscle phase.

Question: *Can I split up the workout into morning and evening sessions?*

Answer: Absolutely. The individual training sessions can be managed in just about any way you desire. If performing double splits (i.e., morning and evening workouts) works best for your lifestyle, go for it; there's no downside to the approach and some (albeit limited) evidence suggests two-a-days may even enhance results. If you choose to do so, remember that nutrient timing takes on greater importance, as discussed in chapter 11. Thus, make sure you consume carbohydrate relatively quickly following your morning training session.

Question: *I'm concerned about adding too much body fat during bulking. Is there any benefit or detriment to doing mini-cuts every month or so?*

Answer: The term "mini-cut" means different things to different people. I'm assuming you're referring to interspersing short periods (two weeks or so) of caloric restriction during a muscle-building diet. I have heard some fitness pros claim that such a strategy facilitates greater muscle gains by enhancing nutrient sensitivity. This may have some validity.

However, while it's technically true that excess body fat can impair cellular signaling, this generally is specific to obesity; I've seen no evidence it occurs in those who maintain reasonable body fat levels. Given that the recommendations laid out in chapter 11 seek to minimize fat gain while maximizing lean mass accretion, it is doubtful that you'd experience any negative effects on cell signaling that would impair gains.

The downside to mini-cuts is that the body is catabolic during periods of caloric restriction, so you'll delay the hypertrophy process during these catabolic periods. On the flip side of the coin, you'll need to diet down eventually if your goal is to get lean, and at that point you'll be in a catabolic state. So ultimately the use of mini-cuts comes down to goals and preferences. If your goal is to maximize growth and you don't mind holding on to a little extra body fat over time, then I wouldn't recommend mini-cuts. Alternatively, if your goal is to maximize growth while getting shredded (i.e., bodybuilding-type goals), you could either opt for employing regimented mini-cuts or simply choose to bulk and then cut; both strategies are viable. If you do decide to implement mini-cuts during the muscle phase of the program, I'd suggest doing so in block 1 when volume is on the lower side; you want to have all your energy and resources available during the higher-volume blocks to maximize the growth response.

Question: *I want to lose weight as well as build muscle. Can I diet down while doing the program? Or is it better to lose weight prior to starting the program and then attempt to add lean mass?*

Answer: You certainly can go through the program with the goal of recomping. Just understand that the strategy will somewhat compromise your muscular gains. As discussed in chapter 11, it's possible to gain muscle during a caloric deficit (a requirement to lose body fat). However, a caloric deficit necessarily puts you in a catabolic state, which is not conducive to adding lean mass. So as long as you understand this conundrum and take the position that losing fat is more important than maximizing hypertrophy, go for it.

I'd also note that you can take advantage of "diet breaks" to help further gains in lean mass. In this strategy, you diet for a given period of time (generally three to six weeks) and then take a break from dieting so calories are increased above maintenance for a short period of time (generally a week or so). Note that although this does help to enhance muscle development and may also have psychological benefits for dietary adherence, it will prolong the time it takes to get down to your goal body fat percentage. So determine whether you're okay with the trade-off.

If you choose to take diet breaks, I'd suggest that you structure your schedule so that a break falls in block 3 of the muscle phase. This will help to support energy levels when training volume is at its highest, as well as provide the necessary caloric requirements for optimal muscle building.

Question: *Can I change the splits in the muscle phase?*

Answer: For sure. The sample routines are simply provided as examples of how you might choose to go about structuring the program. You can split your routine in numerous ways; there is no universal "best" body part split. Consider your body's strengths and weaknesses when deciding on a split. You might want to increase the frequency of training for a lagging muscle group, which could necessitate altering the split so that muscles get adequate recovery between sessions. The art of exercise program design requires careful consideration of your individual needs in concert with the principles of exercise science; make sure you take both factors into account.

Question: *The sample routine in the final block of the muscle phase lasts only two weeks. Can I extend it?*

Answer: As mentioned throughout the book, the program should be considered a template for hypertrophy program design rather than a rigid workout plan; you are encouraged to customize it to your individual needs, abilities, and preferences. Understand, though, that the final hypertrophy block is designed to push your body to its limits in an effort to promote functional overreaching. When done properly, this elicits a supercompensatory response that maximizes muscle growth. However, push your body too far and you'll end up overtrained, which has a detrimental effect on gains.

In my experience, a two-week block is a good duration for most people; rarely will this push someone over the edge and into an overtrained state. That said, responses vary, and some are able to prosper with an extra week or even two in block 3. If you're highly experienced and know your body well enough to believe that you can handle the additional stress, then by all means give it a go. Just be cognizant of how you feel on a day-to-day basis. In particular, pay attention to the manifestation of symptoms of overtraining, as discussed in chapter 2. When in doubt, opt to cut the block short; the possibility of becoming overtrained and its associated detrimental effects on your body simply isn't worth the risk.

Question: *I train in a busy gym and it's difficult to set up the supersets and circuit training schemes recommended during the metabolic phase. Is there anything I can do?*

Answer: Training in a gym is often a challenge with respect to equipment availability. Of course you need to be respectful of the needs of others and cannot impede their ability to work out. If the gym is crowded, you probably won't be able to move quickly between machines, thus negating the utility of supersets and circuit training.

One solution is to modify the exercise selection by using dumbbells. Depending on how well-stocked your gym is, you should be able to gather the needed dumbbells in a secluded area of the gym and go through the routine. If not, then simply perform the routine in straight sets, as described in the first microcycle. It's not ideal, but the overall effect on your results will be relatively minor.

Question: *Is there a reason you don't you include deadlifts in the sample routines during the muscle phase? I like to deadlift!*

Answer: While deadlifts are an excellent exercise for developing strength, I personally don't feel they are a particularly good choice during a cycle of hypertrophy-focused training. The issue here is that the deadlift substantially taxes the neuromuscular system over and above that of other exercises. Hence, it saps recovery, hindering your ability to tolerate the higher volumes of training during the muscle phase. Moreover, a majority of the body's total musculature is involved in performance, making it difficult to structure your split when training four or more days per week. All things considered, the risks outweigh the rewards in my humble opinion, particularly given that there are alternatives without the corresponding downside; there certainly is no reason that deadlifts must be included to maximize hypertrophy.

That said, you're certainly welcome to integrate deadlifts into the routine. Training should be fun, and if you really like performing deadlifts, then that's reason enough to keep them as a staple exercise. Just be aware of the issues I mentioned. If you're not recovering as well as you should, it may well be from the inclusion of the deadlift. Always be objective in assessing your training evolution and open to reevaluating your choices and alternatives if you are not progressing in a consistent manner.

Question: *Is there a best time of day to train to maximize growth?*

Answer: The short answer is no. Although some fitness pros claim it's better to train later in the day, this speculation is based on short-term studies that don't necessarily reflect long-term adaptations. It's true that most people are stronger at baseline when tested in the evening. However, the body is highly adaptive. If you consistently train in the morning, your body gets used to this timing and strength levels ultimately become equal to that achieved later in the day. In the same way, increases in muscle size are similar regardless of when you train, provided you consistently work out at the same time.

Thus, the takeaway is that you can train whenever it is preferable and most convenient; there is no need to unduly alter your schedule in quest of greater gains. That said, you should take into account lifestyle factors. If you have a very demanding job, training after work may not be ideal because you'll be sapped of energy to the extent that your gym performance suffers. Alternatively, if you go to work very early, it might be counterproductive to wake up even earlier just to get to the gym; you'll likely be dragging yourself through workouts. Regardless, it's generally best to be consistent in the timing of your workouts. As mentioned, the body is proficient at adapting to training at a given time of day, but if you sometimes train early and other times train late, the adaptation process is short-circuited, which in turn can interfere with results.

Question: *What should I do after completing all phases of the program?*

Answer: The M.A.X. Muscle Plan is designed to be repeated over and over. Once you finish all phases of the program, simply restart the strength phase and proceed through each subsequent phase as you did previously. In fact, you should be able to tweak the program the second time around (and conceivably on subsequent performances as well) to best suit your needs and abilities. In this way, some lifters are able to attain even better results when the program is repeated by gaining insight into their response to training and nutrition and customizing the corresponding variables accordingly.

REFERENCES

Chapter 1

1. Bamman, MM, Roberts, BM, and Adams, GR. Molecular regulation of exercise-induced muscle fiber hypertrophy. *Cold Spring Harb Perspect Med* 8: a029751, 2018. doi:10.1101/cshperspect.a029751.

2. Barton-Davis, ER, Shoturma, DI, and Sweeney, HL. Contribution of satellite cells to IGF-I induced hypertrophy of skeletal muscle. *Acta Physiol Scand* 167: 301-305, 1999.

3. Goldspink, G. Mechanical signals, IGF-I gene splicing, and muscle adaptation. *Physiology (Bethesda)* 20: 232-238, 2005.

4. Harridge, SD. Plasticity of human skeletal muscle: Gene expression to in vivo function. *Exp Physiol* 92: 783-797, 2007.

5. Kakehi, S, Tamura, Y, Kubota, A, Takeno, K, Kawaguchi, M, Sakuraba, K, Kawamori, R, and Watada, H. Effects of blood flow restriction on muscle size and gene expression in muscle during immobilization: A pilot study. *Physiol Rep* 8: e14516, 2020.

6. Kim, JS, Petrella, JK, Cross, JM, and Bamman, MM. Load-mediated downregulation of myostatin mRNA is not sufficient to promote myofiber hypertrophy in humans: A cluster analysis. *J Appl Physiol (1985)* 103: 1488-1495, 2007.

7. Lang, F, Busch, GL, Ritter, M, Volkl, H, Waldegger, S, Gulbins, E, and Haussinger, D. Functional significance of cell volume regulatory mechanisms. *Physiol Rev* 78: 247-306, 1998.

8. Lasevicius, T, Ugrinowitsch, C, Schoenfeld, BJ, Roschel, H, Tavares, LD, De Souza, EO, Laurentino, G, and Tricoli, V. Effects of different intensities of resistance training with equated volume load on muscle strength and hypertrophy. *Eur J Sport Sci* 18: 772-780, 2018.

9. Lixandrao, ME, Ugrinowitsch, C, Berton, R, Vechin, FC, Conceicao, MS, Damas, F, Libardi, CA, and Roschel, H. Magnitude of muscle strength and mass adaptations between high-load resistance training versus low-load resistance training associated with blood-flow restriction: A systematic review and meta-analysis. *Sports Med* 48: 361-378, 2018.

10. McHugh, MP. Recent advances in the understanding of the repeated bout effect: The protective effect against muscle damage from a single bout of eccentric exercise. *Scand J Med Sci Sports* 13: 88-97, 2003.

11. Morton, RW, Sato, K, Gallaugher, MPB, Oikawa, SY, McNicholas, PD, Fujita, S, and Phillips, SM. Muscle androgen receptor content but not systemic hormones is associated with resistance training-induced skeletal muscle hypertrophy in healthy, young men. *Front Physiol* 9: 1373, 2018.

12. Moss, FP, and Leblond, CP. Satellite cells as the source of nuclei in muscles of growing rats. *Anat Rec* 170: 421-435, 1971.

13. Perez-Lopez, A, McKendry, J, Martin-Rincon, M, Morales-Alamo, D, Perez-Kohler, B, Valades, D, Bujan, J, Calbet, JAL, and Breen, L. Skeletal muscle IL-15/IL-15Rα and myofibrillar protein synthesis after resistance exercise. *Scand J Med Sci Sports* 28: 116-125, 2018.

14. Petrella, JK, Kim, J, Mayhew, DL, Cross, JM, and Bamman, MM. Potent myofiber hypertrophy during resistance training in humans is associated with satellite cell-mediated myonuclear addition: A cluster analysis. *J Appl Physiol* 104: 1736-1742, 2008.

15. Schoenfeld, BJ. The mechanisms of muscle hypertrophy and their application to resistance training. *J Strength Cond Res* 24: 2857-2872, 2010.

16. Schoenfeld, BJ. Does exercise-induced muscle damage play a role in skeletal muscle hypertrophy? *J Strength Cond Res* 26: 1441-1453, 2012.

17. Schoenfeld, BJ. Postexercise hypertrophic adaptations: A reexamination of the hormone hypothesis and its applicability to resistance training program design. *J Strength Cond Res* 27: 1720-1730, 2013.

18. Schoenfeld, BJ, Ratamess, NA, Peterson, MD, Contreras, B, Tiryaki-Sonmez, G, and Alvar, BA. Effects of different volume-equated resistance training loading strategies on muscular adaptations in well-trained men. *J Strength Cond Res* 28: 2909-2918, 2014.

19. Schoenfeld, BJ, Ogborn, DI, and Krieger, JW. Effect of repetition duration during resistance training on muscle hypertrophy: A systematic review and meta-analysis. *Sports Med* 45: 577-585, 2015.

20. Schoenfeld, BJ, Grgic, J, Ogborn, D, and Krieger, JW. Strength and hypertrophy adaptations between low- vs. high-load resistance training: A systematic review and meta-analysis. *J Strength Cond Res* 31: 3508-3523, 2017.

21. Sculthorpe, N, Solomon, AM, Sinanan, AC, Bouloux, PM, Grace, F, and Lewis, MP. Androgens affect myogenesis in vitro and increase local IGF-1 expression. *Med Sci Sports Exerc* 44: 610-615, 2012.

22. Sinha-Hikim, I, Cornford, M, Gaytan, H, Lee, ML, and Bhasin, S. Effects of testosterone supplementation on skeletal muscle fiber hypertrophy and satellite cells in community-dwelling older men. *J Clin Endocrinol Metab* 91: 3024-3033, 2006.

23. Spangenburg, EE. Changes in muscle mass with mechanical load: Possible cellular mechanisms. *Appl Physiol Nutr Metab* 34: 328-335, 2009.

24. Urban, RJ, Bodenburg, YH, Gilkison, C, Foxworth, J, Coggan, AR, Wolfe, RR, and Ferrando, A. Testosterone administration to elderly men increases skeletal muscle strength and protein synthesis. *Am J Physiol* 269: E820-E826, 1995.

25. Velloso, CP. Regulation of muscle mass by growth hormone and IGF-I. *Br J Pharmacol* 154: 557-568, 2008.

26. Wackerhage, H, Schoenfeld, BJ, Hamilton, DL, Lehti, M, and Hulmi, JJ. Stimuli and sensors that initiate skeletal muscle hypertrophy following resistance exercise. *J Appl Physiol (1985)* 126: 30-43, 2019.

27. Zhao, W, Pan, J, Zhao, Z, Wu, Y, Bauman, WA, and Cardozo, CP. Testosterone protects against dexamethasone-induced muscle atrophy, protein degradation and MAFbx upregulation. *J Steroid Biochem Mol Biol* 110: 125-129, 2008.

Chapter 2

1. Adams, G, and Bamman, MM. Characterization and regulation of mechanical loading-induced compensatory muscle hypertrophy. *Comprehensive Physiology* 2829, 2012.

2. Behm, DG, Anderson, K, and Curnew, RS. Muscle force and activation under stable and unstable conditions. *J Strength Cond Res* 16: 416-422, 2002.

3. Carlson, L, Jonker, B, Westcott, WL, Steele, J, and Fisher, JP. Neither repetition duration nor number of muscle actions affect strength increases, body composition, muscle size, or fasted blood glucose in trained males and females. *Appl Physiol Nutr Metab* 44: 200-207, 2019.

4. Colquhoun, RJ, Gai, CM, Aguilar, D, Bove, D, Dolan, J, Vargas, A, Couvillion, K, Jenkins, NDM, and Campbell, BI. Training volume, not frequency, indicative of maximal strength adaptations to resistance training. *J Strength Cond Res* 32: 1207-1213, 2018.

5. Figueiredo, VC, de Salles, BF, and Trajano, GS. Volume for muscle hypertrophy and health outcomes: The most effective variable in resistance training. *Sports Med* 48: 499-505, 2018.

6. Franchi, MV, Atherton, PJ, Reeves, ND, Fluck, M, Williams, J, Mitchell, WK, Selby, A, Beltran Valls, RM, and Narici, MV. Architectural, functional and molecular responses to concentric and eccentric loading in human skeletal muscle. *Acta Physiol (Oxf)* 210: 642-654, 2014.

7. Grgic, J, Lazinica, B, Mikulic, P, Krieger, JW, and Schoenfeld, BJ. The effects of short versus long inter-set rest intervals in resistance training on measures of muscle hypertrophy: A systematic review. *Eur J Sport Sci* 17: 983-993, 2017.

8. Grgic, J, and Schoenfeld, BJ. Are the hypertrophic adaptations to high and low-load resistance training muscle fiber type specific? *Front Physiol* 9: 402, 2018.

9. Grgic, J, Schoenfeld, BJ, Davies, TB, Lazinica, B, Krieger, JW, and Pedisic, Z. Effect of resistance training frequency on gains in muscular strength: A systematic review and meta-analysis. *Sports Med* 48: 1207-1220, 2018.

10. Hammarstrom, D, Ofsteng, S, Koll, L, Hanestadhaugen, M, Hollan, I, Apro, W, Whist, JE, Blomstrand, E, Ronnestad, BR, and Ellefsen, S. Benefits of higher resistance-training volume are related to ribosome biogenesis. *J Physiol* 598: 543-565, 2019.

11. Helms, ER, Cronin, J, Storey, A, and Zourdos, MC. Application of the repetitions in reserve-based rating of perceived exertion scale for resistance training. *Strength Cond J* 38: 42-49, 2016.

12. Izquierdo, M, Ibanez, J, Gonzalez-Badillo, JJ, Hakkinen, K, Ratamess, NA, Kraemer, WJ, French, DN, Eslava, J, Altadill, A, Asiain, X, and Gorostiaga, EM. Differential effects of strength training leading to failure versus not to failure on hormonal responses, strength, and muscle power gains. *J Appl Physiol* 100: 1647-1656, 2006.

13. Ormsbee, MJ, Carzoli, JP, Klemp, A, Allman, BR, Zourdos, MC, Kim, JS, and Panton, LB. Efficacy of the repetitions in reserve-based rating of perceived exertion for the bench press in experienced and novice benchers. *J Strength Cond Res* 33: 337-345, 2019.

14. Saric, J, Lisica, D, Orlic, I, Grgic, J, Krieger, JW, Vuk, S, and Schoenfeld, BJ. Resistance training frequencies of 3 and 6 times per week produce similar muscular adaptations in resistance-trained men. *J Strength Cond Res* 33: S122-S129, 2018. doi:10.1519/JSC.0000000000002909.

15. Schoenfeld, BJ. Postexercise hypertrophic adaptations: A reexamination of the hormone hypothesis and its applicability to resistance training program design. *J Strength Cond Res* 27: 1720-1730, 2013.

16. Schoenfeld, BJ, Ogborn, DI, and Krieger, JW. Effect of repetition duration during resistance training on muscle hypertrophy: A systematic review and meta-analysis. *Sports Med* 45: 577-585, 2015.

17. Schoenfeld, BJ, Grgic, J, Ogborn, D, and Krieger, JW. Strength and hypertrophy adaptations between low- vs. high-load resistance training: A systematic review and meta-analysis. *J Strength Cond Res* 31: 3508-3523, 2017.

18. Schoenfeld, BJ, Ogborn, D, and Krieger, JW. Dose-response relationship between weekly resistance training volume and increases in muscle mass: A systematic review and meta-analysis. *J Sports Sci* 35: 1073-1082, 2017.

19. Schoenfeld, BJ, Ogborn, DI, Vigotsky, AD, Franchi, MV, and Krieger, JW. Hypertrophic effects of concentric vs. eccentric muscle actions: A systematic review and meta-analysis. *J Strength Cond Res* 31: 2599-2608, 2017.

20. Schoenfeld, BJ, Grgic, J, and Krieger, J. How many times per week should a muscle be trained to maximize muscle hypertrophy? A systematic review and meta-analysis of studies examining the effects of resistance training frequency. *J Sports Sci* 37: 1286-1295, 2019.

21. Schoenfeld, BJ, Vigotsky, AD, Grgic, J, Haun, C, Contreras, B, Delcastillo, K, Francis, A, Cote, G, and Alto, A. Do the anatomical and physiological properties of a muscle determine its adaptive response to different loading protocols? *Physiol Rep* 8: e14427, 2020.

22. Schuenke, MD, Herman, JR, Gliders, RM, Hagerman, FC, Hikida, RS, Rana, SR, Ragg, KE, and Staron, RS. Early-phase muscular adaptations in response to slow-speed versus traditional resistance-training regimens. *Eur J Appl Physiol* 112: 3585-3595, 2012.

23. Senna, GW, Figueiredo, T, Scudese, E, Baffi, M, Carneiro, F, Moraes, E, Miranda, H, and Simão, R. Influence of different rest interval lengths in multi-joint and single-joint exercises on repetition performance, perceived exertion, and blood lactate. *J Exerc Physiol* 15: 96-106, 2012.

24. Sternlicht, E, Rugg, S, Fujii, LL, Tomomitsu, KF, and Seki, MM. Electromyographic comparison of a stability ball crunch with a traditional crunch. *J Strength Cond Res* 21: 506-509, 2007.

25. Walsh, NP, Blannin, AK, Robson, PJ, and Gleeson, M. Glutamine, exercise and immune function: Links and possible mechanisms. *Sports Med* 26: 177-191, 1998.

26. Wulf, G. Attentional focus and motor learning: A review of 15 years. *International Review of Sport and Exercise Psychology* 6: 77-104, 2013.

Chapter 6

1. Henschke, N, and Lin, CC. Stretching before or after exercise does not reduce delayed-onset muscle soreness. *Br J Sports Med* 45: 1249-1250, 2011.

2. Morton, SK, Whitehead, JR, Brinkert, RH, and Caine, DJ. Resistance training vs. static stretching: Effects on flexibility and strength. *J Strength Cond Res* 25: 3391-3398, 2011.

3. Ribeiro, AS, Romanzini, M, Schoenfeld, BJ, Souza, MF, Avelar, A, and Cyrino, ES. Effect of different warm-up procedures on the performance of resistance training exercises. *Percept Mot Skills* 119: 133-145, 2014.

4. Rubini, EC, Costa, AL, and Gomes, PS. The effects of stretching on strength performance. *Sports Med* 37: 213-224, 2007.

5. Thacker, SB, Gilchrist, J, Stroup, DF, and Kimsey, CD, Jr. The impact of stretching on sports injury risk: A systematic review of the literature. *Med Sci Sports Exerc* 36: 371-378, 2004.

Chapter 8

1. Davies, T, Orr, R, Halaki, M, and Hackett, D. Effect of training leading to repetition failure on muscular strength: A systematic review and meta-analysis. *Sports Med* 46: 487-502, 2016.

2. De Luca, CJ, and Contessa, P. Hierarchical control of motor units in voluntary contractions. *J Neurophysiol* 107: 178-195, 2012.

3. Escamilla, RF, Fleisig, GS, Zheng, N, Lander, JE, Barrentine, SW, Andrews, JR, Bergemann, BW, and Moorman, CT, 3rd. Effects of technique variations on knee biomechanics during the squat and leg press. *Med Sci Sports Exerc* 33: 1552-1566, 2001.

4. Kukulka, CG, and Clamann, HP. Comparison of the recruitment and discharge properties of motor units in human brachial biceps and adductor pollicis during isometric contractions. *Brain Res* 219: 45-55, 1981.

5. Schoenfeld, BJ, Peterson, MD, Ogborn, D, Contreras, B, and Sonmez, GT. Effects of low- versus high-load resistance training on muscle strength and hypertrophy in well-trained men. *J Strength Cond Res* 29: 2954-2963, 2015.

6. Schoenfeld, BJ, Contreras, B, Krieger, J, Grgic, J, Delcastillo, K, Belliard, R, and Alto, A. Resistance training volume enhances muscle hypertrophy but not strength in trained men. *Med Sci Sports Exerc* 51: 94-103, 2019.

Chapter 9

1. de Freitas Maia, M, Paz, GA, Miranda, H, Lima, V, Bentes, CM, da Silva Novaes, J, Dos Santos Vigário, P, and Willardson, JM. Maximal repetition performance, rating of perceived exertion, and muscle fatigue during paired set training performed with different rest intervals. *J Exerc Sci Fit* 13: 104-110, 2015.

2. Farinatti, PT, and Castinheiras Neto, AG. The effect of between-set rest intervals on the oxygen uptake during and after resistance exercise sessions performed with large- and small-muscle mass. *J Strength Cond Res* 25: 3181-3190, 2011.

3. Fry, AC. The role of resistance exercise intensity on muscle fibre adaptations. *Sports Med* 34: 663-679, 2004.

4. Grgic, J, and Schoenfeld, BJ. Are the hypertrophic adaptations to high and low-load resistance training muscle fiber type specific? *Front Physiol* 9: 402, 2018.

5. Ohno, Y, Ando, K, Ito, T, Suda, Y, Matsui, Y, Oyama, A, Kaneko, H, Yokoyama, S, Egawa, T, and Goto, K. Lactate stimulates a potential for hypertrophy and regeneration of mouse skeletal muscle. *Nutrients* 11: 869, 2019. doi:10.3390/nu11040869.

6. Oishi, Y, Tsukamoto, H, Yokokawa, T, Hirotsu, K, Shimazu, M, Uchida, K, Tomi, H, Higashida, K, Iwanaka, N, and Hashimoto, T. Mixed lactate and caffeine compound increases satellite cell activity and anabolic signals for muscle hypertrophy. *J Appl Physiol (1985)* 118: 742-749, 2015.

7. Tsukamoto, S, Shibasaki, A, Naka, A, Saito, H, and Iida, K. Lactate promotes myoblast differentiation and myotube hypertrophy via a pathway involving MyoD in vitro and enhances muscle regeneration in vivo. *Int J Mol Sci* 19: 3649, 2018. doi:10.3390/ijms19113649.

Chapter 10

1. Angleri, V, Ugrinowitsch, C, and Libardi, CA. Crescent pyramid and drop-set systems do not promote greater strength gains, muscle hypertrophy, and changes on muscle architecture compared with traditional resistance training in well-trained men. *Eur J Appl Physiol* 117: 359-369, 2017.

2. Antonio, J, and Gonyea, WJ. Progressive stretch overload of skeletal muscle results in hypertrophy before hyperplasia. *J Appl Physiol (1985)* 75: 1263-1271, 1993.

3. Fink, J, Schoenfeld, BJ, Kikuchi, N, and Nakazato, K. Effects of drop set resistance training on acute stress indicators and long-term muscle hypertrophy and strength. *J Sports Med Phys Fitness* 58: 597-605, 2017.

4. Hody, S, Croisier, JL, Bury, T, Rogister, B, and Leprince, P. Eccentric muscle contractions: Risks and benefits. *Front Physiol* 10: 536, 2019.

5. Nunes, JP, Grgic, J, Cunha, PM, Ribeiro, AS, Schoenfeld, BJ, de Salles, BF, and Cyrino, ES. What influence does resistance exercise order have on muscular strength gains and muscle hypertrophy? A systematic review and meta-analysis. *Eur J Sport Sci* 21: 149-157, 2021.

6. Silva, JE, Lowery, RP, Antonio, J, McClearly, S, Rauch, J, Ormes, J, Shields, K, Sharp, M, Georges, J, Weiner, S, Joy, J, and Wilson, JM. Weighted post-set stretching increases skeletal muscle hypertrophy (NSCA 2014 annual meeting). *J Strength Cond Res* 28: 65, 2014.

7. Simpson, CL, Kim, BDH, Bourcet, MR, Jones, GR, and Jakobi, JM. Stretch training induces unequal adaptation in muscle fascicles and thickness in medial and lateral gastrocnemii. *Scand J Med Sci Sports* 27: 1597-1604, 2017.

Chapter 11

1. Antonio, J, Peacock, CA, Ellerbroek, A, Fromhoff, B, and Silver, T. The effects of consuming a high protein diet (4.4 g/kg/d) on body composition in resistance-trained individuals. *J Int Soc Sports Nutr* 11: 19, 2014.

2. Antonio, J, Ellerbroek, A, Silver, T, Orris, S, Scheiner, M, Gonzalez, A, and Peacock, CA. A high protein diet (3.4 g/kg/d) combined with a heavy resistance training program improves body composition in healthy trained men and women: A follow-up investigation. *J Int Soc Sports Nutr* 12: 39, 2015.

3. Aragon, AA, and Schoenfeld, BJ. Magnitude and composition of the energy surplus for maximizing muscle hypertrophy: Implications for bodybuilding and physique athletes. *Strength Cond J* 42: 79-86, 2020.

4. Aragon, AA, and Schoenfeld, BJ. Nutrient timing revisited: Is there a post-exercise anabolic window? *J Int Soc Sports Nutr* 10: 5, 2013.

5. Areta, JL, Burke, LM, Ross, ML, Camera, DM, West, DW, Broad, EM, Jeacocke, NA, Moore, DR, Stellingwerff, T, Phillips, SM, Hawley, JA, and Coffey, VG. Timing and distribution of protein ingestion during prolonged recovery from resistance exercise alters myofibrillar protein synthesis. *J Physiol* 591: 2319-2331, 2013.

6. Bandegan, A, Courtney-Martin, G, Rafii, M, Pencharz, PB, and Lemon, PW. Indicator amino acid-derived estimate of dietary protein requirement for male bodybuilders on a nontraining day is several-fold greater than the current recommended dietary allowance. *J Nutr* 147: 850-857, 2017.

7. Berardi, JM, Price, TB, Noreen, EE, and Lemon, PW. Postexercise muscle glycogen recovery enhanced with a carbohydrate-protein supplement. *Med Sci Sports Exerc* 38: 1106-1113, 2006.

8. Bilsborough, S, and Mann, N. A review of issues of dietary protein intake in humans. *Int J Sport Nutr Exerc Metab* 16: 129-152, 2006.

9. Biolo, G, Williams, BD, Fleming, RY, and Wolfe, RR. Insulin action on muscle protein kinetics and amino acid transport during recovery after resistance exercise. *Diabetes* 48: 949-957, 1999.

10. Burd, NA, West, DW, Moore, DR, Atherton, PJ, Staples, AW, Prior, T, Tang, JE, Rennie, MJ, Baker, SK, and Phillips, SM. Enhanced amino acid sensitivity of myofibrillar protein synthesis persists for up to 24 h after resistance exercise in young men. *J Nutr* 141: 568-573, 2011.

11. Campbell, BI, Aguilar, D, Conlin, L, Vargas, A, Schoenfeld, BJ, Corson, A, Gai, C, Best, S, Galvan, E, and Couvillion, K. Effects of high versus low protein intake on body composition and maximal strength in aspiring female physique athletes engaging in an 8-week resistance training program. *Int J Sport Nutr Exerc Metab* 28: 580-585, 2018.

12. Carbone, JW, McClung, JP, and Pasiakos, SM. Skeletal muscle responses to negative energy balance: Effects of dietary protein. *Adv Nutr* 3: 119-126, 2012.

13. Devries, MC, Sithamparapillai, A, Brimble, KS, Banfield, L, Morton, RW, and Phillips, SM. Changes in kidney function do not differ between healthy adults consuming higher- compared with lower- or normal-protein diets: A systematic review and meta-analysis. *J Nutr* 148: 1760-1775, 2018.

14. Fox, AK, Kaufman, AE, and Horowitz, JF. Adding fat calories to meals after exercise does not alter glucose tolerance. *J Appl Physiol* 97: 11-16, 2004.

15. Garthe, I, Raastad, T, Refsnes, PE, and Sundgot-Borgen, J. Effect of nutritional intervention on body composition and performance in elite athletes. *Eur J Sport Sci* 13: 295-303, 2013.

16. Gorissen, SH, Burd, NA, Hamer, HM, Gijsen, AP, Groen, BB, and van Loon, LJ. Carbohydrate coingestion delays dietary protein digestion and absorption but does not modulate postprandial muscle protein accretion. *J Clin Endocrinol Metab* 99: 2250-2258, 2014.

17. Gropper, SS, Smith, JL, and Groff, JL. *Advanced Nutrition and Human Metabolism.* Belmont, CA: Wadsworth Cengage Learning, 2009.

18. Hainault, I, Carolotti, M, Hajduch, E, Guichard, C, and Lavau, M. Fish oil in a high lard diet prevents obesity, hyperlipemia, and adipocyte insulin resistance in rats. *Ann N Y Acad Sci* 683: 98-101, 1993.

19. Hall, KD, Ayuketah, A, Brychta, R, Cai, H, Cassimatis, T, Chen, KY, Chung, ST, Costa, E, Courville, A, Darcey, V, Fletcher, LA, Forde, CG, Gharib, AM, Guo, J, Howard, R, Joseph, PV, McGehee, S, Ouwerkerk, R, Raisinger, K, Rozga, I, Stagliano, M, Walter, M, Walter, PJ, Yang, S, and Zhou, M. Ultra-processed diets cause excess calorie intake and weight gain: An inpatient randomized controlled trial of ad libitum food intake. *Cell Metab* 30: 67-77.e3, 2019.

20. Hamer, HM, Wall, BT, Kiskini, A, de Lange, A, Groen, BB, Bakker, JA, Gijsen, AP, Verdijk, LB, and van Loon, LJ. Carbohydrate co-ingestion with protein does not further augment post-prandial muscle protein accretion in older men. *Nutr Metab (Lond)* 10: 15, 2013.

21. Hepburn, D, and Maughan, RJ. Glycogen availability as a limiting factor in the performance of isometric exercise. *J Physiol* 342: 52P-53P, 1982.

22. Hulmi, JJ, Laakso, M, Mero, AA, Hakkinen, K, Ahtiainen, JP, and Peltonen, H. The effects of whey protein with or without carbohydrates on resistance training adaptations. *J Int Soc Sports Nutr* 12: 48, 2015.

23. Ivy, J, and Portman, R. *Nutrient Timing: The Future of Sports Nutrition.* North Bergen, NJ: Basic Health Publications, 2004.

24. Ivy, JL. Glycogen resynthesis after exercise: Effect of carbohydrate intake. *Int J Sports Med* 19: S142-S145, 1998.

25. Jacquet, P, Schutz, Y, Montani, JP, and Dulloo, A. How dieting might make some fatter: Modeling weight cycling toward obesity from a perspective of body composition autoregulation. *Int J Obes (Lond)* 44: 1243-1253, 2020.

26. Kerksick, C, Harvey, T, Stout, J, Campbell, B, Wilborn, C, Kreider, R, Kalman, D, Ziegenfuss, T, Lopez, H, Landis, J, Ivy, JL, and Antonio, J. International Society of Sports Nutrition position stand: Nutrient timing. *J Int Soc Sports Nutr* 5: 17, 2008.

27. Kim, IY, Schutzler, S, Schrader, A, Spencer, HJ, Azhar, G, Ferrando, AA, and Wolfe, RR. The anabolic response to a meal containing different amounts of protein is not limited by the maximal stimulation of protein synthesis in healthy young adults. *Am J Physiol Endocrinol Metab* 310: E73-E80, 2016.

28. Koopman, R, Beelen, M, Stellingwerff, T, Pennings, B, Saris, WH, Kies, AK, Kuipers, H, and van Loon, LJ. Coingestion of carbohydrate with protein does not further augment postexercise muscle protein synthesis. *Am J Physiol Endocrinol Metab* 293: E833-E842, 2007.

29. Lambert, CP, and Flynn, MG. Fatigue during high-intensity intermittent exercise: Application to bodybuilding. *Sports Med* 32: 511-522, 2002.

30. Langfort, J, Zarzeczny, R, Pilis, W, Nazar, K, and Kaciuba-Uscitko, H. The effect of a low-carbohydrate diet on performance, hormonal and metabolic responses to a 30-s bout of supramaximal exercise. *Eur J Appl Physiol Occup Physiol* 76: 128-133, 1997.

31. Larson, DE, Tataranni, PA, Ferraro, RT, and Ravussin, E. Ad libitum food intake on a "cafeteria diet" in Native American women: Relations with body composition and 24-h energy expenditure. *Am J Clin Nutr* 62: 911-917, 1995.

32. Layman, DK. Protein quantity and quality at levels above the RDA improves adult weight loss. *J Am Coll Nutr* 23: 631S-636S, 2004.

33. Leveritt, M, and Abernethy, PJ. Effects of carbohydrate restriction on strength performance. *J Strength Cond Res* 13: 52-57, 1999.

34. Lima-Silva, AE, Pires, FO, Bertuzzi, R, Silva-Cavalcante, MD, Oliveira, RS, Kiss, MA, and Bishop, D. Effects of a low- or a high-carbohydrate diet on performance, energy system contribution, and metabolic responses during supramaximal exercise. *Appl Physiol Nutr Metab* 38: 928-934, 2013.

35. Longland, TM, Oikawa, SY, Mitchell, CJ, Devries, MC, and Phillips, SM. Higher compared with lower dietary protein during an energy deficit combined with intense exercise promotes greater lean mass gain and fat mass loss: A randomized trial. *Am J Clin Nutr* 103: 738-746, 2016.

36. Macnaughton, LS, Wardle, SL, Witard, OC, McGlory, C, Hamilton, DL, Jeromson, S, Lawrence, CE, Wallis, GA, and Tipton, KD. The response of muscle protein synthesis following whole-body resistance exercise is greater following 40 g than 20 g of ingested whey protein. *Physiol Rep* 4: e12893, 2016. doi:10.14814/phy2.12893.

37. Mifflin, MD, St Jeor, ST, Hill, LA, Scott, BJ, Daugherty, SA, and Koh, YO. A new predictive equation for resting energy expenditure in healthy individuals. *Am J Clin Nutr* 51: 241-247, 1990.

38. Mitchell, JB, DiLauro, PC, Pizza, FX, and Cavender, DL. The effect of preexercise carbohydrate status on resistance exercise performance. *Int J Sport Nutr* 7: 185-196, 1997.

39. Mohr, AE, Jäger, R, Carpenter, KC, Kerksick, CM, Purpura, M, Townsend, JR, West, NP, Black, K, Gleeson, M, Pyne, DB, Wells, SD, Arent, SM, Kreider, RB, Campbell, BI, Bannock, L, Scheiman, J, Wissent, CJ, Pane, M, Kalman, DS, Pugh, JN, Ortega-

Santos, CP, Ter Haar, JA, Arciero, PJ, and Antonio, J. The athletic gut microbiota. *J Int Soc Sports Nutr* 17: 24, 2020.

40. Moro, T, Tinsley, G, Bianco, A, Marcolin, G, Pacelli, QF, Battaglia, G, Palma, A, Gentil, P, Neri, M, and Paoli, A. Effects of eight weeks of time-restricted feeding (16/8) on basal metabolism, maximal strength, body composition, inflammation, and cardiovascular risk factors in resistance-trained males. *J Transl Med* 14: 290, 2016.

41. Müller, MJ, Geisler, C, Heymsfield, SB, and Bosy-Westphal, A. Recent advances in understanding body weight homeostasis in humans. *F1000Res* 7, 2018. doi:10.12688/f1000research.14151.1.

42. Okuno, M, Kajiwara, K, Imai, S, Kobayashi, T, Honma, N, Maki, T, Suruga, K, Goda, T, Takase, S, Muto, Y, and Moriwaki, H. Perilla oil prevents the excessive growth of visceral adipose tissue in rats by down-regulating adipocyte differentiation. *J Nutr* 127: 1752-1757, 1997.

43. Parkin, JA, Carey, MF, Martin, IK, Stojanovska, L, and Febbraio, MA. Muscle glycogen storage following prolonged exercise: Effect of timing of ingestion of high glycemic index food. *Med Sci Sports Exerc* 29: 220-224, 1997.

44. Pasiakos, SM, Vislocky, LM, Carbone, JW, Altieri, N, Konopelski, K, Freake, HC, Anderson, JM, Ferrando, AA, Wolfe, RR, and Rodriguez, NR. Acute energy deprivation affects skeletal muscle protein synthesis and associated intracellular signaling proteins in physically active adults. *J Nutr* 140: 745-751, 2010.

45. Power, O, Hallihan, A, and Jakeman, P. Human insulinotropic response to oral ingestion of native and hydrolysed whey protein. *Amino Acids* 37: 333-339, 2009.

46. Ribeiro, AS, Nunes, JP, Schoenfeld, BJ, Aguiar, AF, and Cyrino, ES. Effects of different dietary energy intake following resistance training on muscle mass and body fat in bodybuilders: A pilot study. *J Hum Kinet* 70: 125-134, 2019. doi:10.2478/hukin-2019-0038.

47. Rivellese, AA, De Natale, C, and Lilli, S. Type of dietary fat and insulin resistance. *Ann N Y Acad Sci* 967: 329-335, 2002.

48. Roberts, RA, Pearson, DR, Costill, DL, Fink, WJ, Pascoe, DD, Benedict, MA, Lambert, CP, and Zachweija, JJ. Muscle glycogenolysis during differing intensities of weight-resistance exercise. *J Appl Physiol* 70: 1700-1706, 1991.

49. Rosqvist, F, Iggman, D, Kullberg, J, Cedernaes, J, Johansson, HE, Larsson, A, Johansson, L, Ahlstrom, H, Arner, P, Dahlman, I, and Riserus, U. Overfeeding polyunsaturated and saturated fat causes distinct effects on liver and visceral fat accumulation in humans. *Diabetes* 63: 2356-2368, 2014.

50. Rozenek, R, Ward, P, Long, S, and Garhammer, J. Effects of high-calorie supplements on body composition and muscular strength following resistance training. *J Sports Med Phys Fitness* 42: 340-347, 2002.

51. Sallinen, J, Pakarinen, A, Ahtiainen, J, Kraemer, WJ, Volek, JS, and Hakkinen, K. Relationship between diet and serum anabolic hormone responses to heavy-resistance exercise in men. *Int J Sports Med* 25: 627-633, 2004.

52. Schoenfeld, BJ, Aragon, AA, and Krieger, JW. The effect of protein timing on muscle strength and hypertrophy: A meta-analysis. *J Int Soc Sports Nutr* 10: 53, 2013.

53. Schoenfeld, BJ, Aragon, A, Wilborn, C, Urbina, SL, Hayward, SE, and Krieger, J. Pre- versus post-exercise protein intake has similar effects on muscular adaptations. *PeerJ* 5: e2825, 2017.

54. Schoenfeld, BJ, and Aragon, AA. How much protein can the body use in a single meal for muscle-building? Implications for daily protein distribution. *J Int Soc Sports Nutr* 15: 10, 2018.

55. Slater, G, and Phillips, SM. Nutrition guidelines for strength sports: Sprinting, weightlifting, throwing events, and bodybuilding. *J Sports Sci* 29: S67-S77, 2011.

56. Staples, AW, Burd, NA, West, DW, Currie, KD, Atherton, PJ, Moore, DR, Rennie, MJ, Macdonald, MJ, Baker, SK, and Phillips, SM. Carbohydrate does not augment exercise-induced protein accretion versus protein alone. *Med Sci Sports Exerc* 43: 1154-1161, 2011.

57. Su, W, and Jones, PJ. Dietary fatty acid composition influences energy accretion in rats. *J Nutr* 123: 2109-2114, 1993.

58. Tchoukalova, YD, Votruba, SB, Tchkonia, T, Giorgadze, N, Kirkland, JL, and Jensen, MD. Regional differences in cellular mechanisms of adipose tissue gain with overfeeding. *Proc Natl Acad Sci U S A* 107: 18226-18231, 2010.

59. Tinsley, GM, Forsse, JS, Butler, NK, Paoli, A, Bane, AA, La Bounty, PM, Morgan, GB, and Grandjean, PW. Time-restricted feeding in young men performing resistance training: A randomized controlled trial. *Eur J Sport Sci* 17: 200-207, 2017.

60. Tinsley, GM, Moore, ML, Graybeal, AJ, Paoli, A, Kim, Y, Gonzales, JU, Harry, JR, VanDusseldorp, TA, Kennedy, DN, and Cruz, MR. Time-restricted feeding plus resistance training in active females: A randomized trial. *Am J Clin Nutr* 110: 628-640, 2019.

61. Volek, JS, Gomez, AL, Love, DM, Avery, NG, Sharman, MJ, and Kraemer, WJ. Effects of a high-fat diet on postabsorptive and postprandial testosterone responses to a fat-rich meal. *Metabolism* 50: 1351-1355, 2001.

62. Wax, B, Kavazis, AN, and Brown, SP. Effects of supplemental carbohydrate ingestion during superimposed electromyostimulation exercise in elite weightlifters. *J Strength Cond Res* 27: 3084-3090, 2013.

63. Yasuda, J, Tomita, T, Arimitsu, T, and Fujita, S. Evenly distributed protein intake over 3 meals augments resistance exercise-induced muscle hypertrophy in healthy young men. *J Nutr* 150: 1845-1851, 2020.

Chapter 12

1. Atherton, PJ, Babraj, J, Smith, K, Singh, J, Rennie, MJ, and Wackerhage, H. Selective activation of AMPK-PGC-1alpha or PKB-TSC2-mTOR signaling can explain specific adaptive responses to endurance or resistance training-like electrical muscle stimulation. *FASEB J* 19: 786-788, 2005.

2. Bloor, CM. Angiogenesis during exercise and training. *Angiogenesis* 8: 263-271, 2005.

3. Coffey, VG, Jemiolo, B, Edge, J, Garnham, AP, Trappe, SW, and Hawley, JA. Effect of consecutive repeated sprint and resistance exercise bouts on acute adaptive responses in human skeletal muscle. *Am J Physiol Regul Integr Comp Physiol* 297: R1441-R1451, 2009.

4. Coffey, VG, Pilegaard, H, Garnham, AP, O'Brien, BJ, and Hawley, JA. Consecutive bouts of diverse contractile activity alter acute responses in human skeletal muscle. *J Appl Physiol (1985)* 106: 1187-1197, 2009.

5. Estes, RR, Malinowski, A, Piacentini, M, Thrush, D, Salley, E, Losey, C, and Hayes, E. The effect of high intensity interval run training on cross-sectional area of the vastus lateralis in untrained college students. *Int J Exerc Sci* 10: 137-145, 2017.

6. Febbraio, MA, Chiu, A, Angus, DJ, Arkinstall, MJ, and Hawley, JA. Effects of carbohydrate ingestion before and during exercise on glucose kinetics and performance. *J Appl Physiol* 89: 2220-2226, 2000.

7. Fyfe, JJ, Bishop, DJ, and Stepto, NK. Interference between concurrent resistance and endurance exercise: Molecular bases and the role of individual training variables. *Sports Med* 44: 743-762, 2014.

8. Goodman, CA, Mayhew, DL, and Hornberger, TA. Recent progress toward understanding the molecular mechanisms that regulate skeletal muscle mass. *Cell Signal* 23: 1896-1906, 2011.

9. Harber, MP, Konopka, AR, Undem, MK, Hinkley, JM, Minchev, K, Kaminsky, LA, Trappe, TA, and Trappe, S. Aerobic exercise training induces skeletal muscle hypertrophy and age-dependent adaptations in myofiber function in young and older men. *J Appl Physiol (1985)* 113: 1495-1504, 2012.

10. Horowitz, JF, Mora-Rodriguez, R, Byerley, LO, and Coyle, EF. Lipolytic suppression following carbohydrate ingestion limits fat oxidation during exercise. *Am J Physiol* 273: E768-E775, 1997.

11. Ismail, I, Keating, SE, Baker, MK, and Johnson, NA. A systematic review and meta-analysis of the effect of aerobic vs. resistance exercise training on visceral fat. *Obes Rev* 13: 68-91, 2012.

12. Laye, MJ, Thyfault, JP, Stump, CS, and Booth, FW. Inactivity induces increases in abdominal fat. *J Appl Physiol (1985)* 102: 1341-1347, 2007.

13. Maestroni, L, Read, P, Bishop, C, Papadopoulos, K, Suchomel, TJ, Comfort, P, and Turner, A. The benefits of strength training on musculoskeletal system health: Practical applications for interdisciplinary care. *Sports Med* 50: 1431-1450, 2020.

14. Mikkola, J, Rusko, H, Izquierdo, M, Gorostiaga, EM, and Hakkinen, K. Neuromuscular and cardiovascular adaptations during concurrent strength and endurance training in untrained men. *Int J Sports Med* 33: 702-710, 2012.

15. Schoenfeld, B. Does cardio after an overnight fast maximize fat loss? *Strength Cond J* 33: 23-25, 2011.

16. Schoenfeld, BJ, Aragon, AA, Wilborn, CD, Krieger, JW, and Sonmez, GT. Body composition changes associated with fasted versus non-fasted aerobic exercise. *J Int Soc Sports Nutr* 11: 54, 2014.

17. Trappe, S, Harber, M, Creer, A, Gallagher, P, Slivka, D, Minchev, K, and Whitsett, D. Single muscle fiber adaptations with marathon training. *J Appl Physiol (1985)* 101: 721-727, 2006.

18. Tsitkanou, S, Spengos, K, Stasinaki, AN, Zaras, N, Bogdanis, G, Papadimas, G, and Terzis, G. Effects of high-intensity interval cycling performed after resistance training on muscle strength and hypertrophy. *Scand J Med Sci Sports* 27: 1317-1327, 2017.

19. Lemon, PW, and Mullin, JP. Effect of initial muscle glycogen levels on protein catabolism during exercise. *J Appl Physiol* 48: 624-629, 1980.

ABOUT THE AUTHOR

Brad Schoenfeld, PhD, CSCS,*D, CSPS,*D, NSCA-CPT,*D, FNSCA, is internationally regarded as one of the foremost authorities on muscle hypertrophy. The 2011 National Strength and Conditioning Association (NSCA) Personal Trainer of the Year, Schoenfeld is a lifetime drug-free bodybuilder who has won multiple natural bodybuilding titles. As a personal trainer, he has worked with numerous elite-level physique athletes, including many top pros.

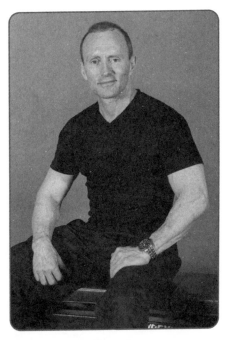

Schoenfeld was the recipient of the 2016 Dwight D. Eisenhower Fitness Award, which is presented by the United States Sports Academy for outstanding achievement in fitness and for contributions to the growth and development of sport fitness through outstanding leadership activity. He was also the 2018 cowinner of the NSCA Outstanding Young Investigator Award. He is the author of multiple books, including *Science and Development of Muscle Hypertrophy* and *Strong & Sculpted*. He has been published or featured in virtually every major fitness magazine and has appeared on hundreds of television shows and radio programs across the United States. Currently, he writes the "Ask the Muscle Doc" column for Bodybuilding.com.

Schoenfeld earned his PhD in health promotion and wellness at Rocky Mountain University, where his research focused on elucidating the mechanisms of muscle hypertrophy and their application to resistance training. He has published more than 300 peer-reviewed scientific papers and serves on the editorial advisory boards for several journals, including the *Journal of Strength and Conditioning Research* and the *Journal of the International Society of Sports Nutrition*.

Schoenfeld is a full professor of exercise science at Lehman College in the Bronx, New York, and is director of the graduate program in human performance and fitness. He previously served as the sports nutrition consultant to the New Jersey Devils hockey organization.

You read the book—now complete the companion CE exam to earn continuing education credit!

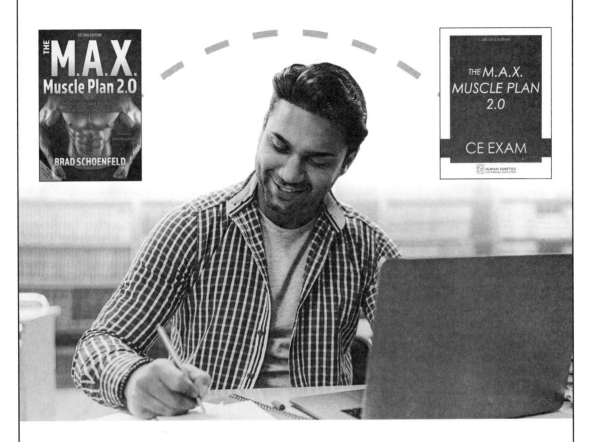

Find and purchase the companion CE exam here:
US.HumanKinetics.com/collections/CE-Exam
Canada.HumanKinetics.com/collections/CE-Exam

50% off the companion CE exam with this code

MMP2022

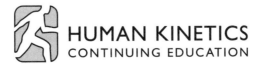

MMP2022
09/21